Beyond Viagra

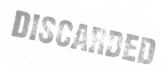

Gerald A. Melchiode, M.D.

with Bill Sloan

An Owl Book
Henry Holt and Company
New York

Beyond

A Commonsense Guide

to Building a Healthy

Sexual Relationship for Both

Men and Women

Viagra

Henry Holt and Company, Inc.
Publishers since 1866
115 West 18th Street
New York, New York 10011

Henry Holt® is a registered trademark of
Henry Holt and Company, Inc.

Published in Canada by Fitzhenry & Whiteside Ltd.,
195 Allstate Parkway, Markham, Ontario L3R 4T8.

Library of Congress Cataloging-in-Publication Data
Melchiode, Gerald A.
Beyond viagra : a commonsense guide to building a
healthy sexual relationship for both men and women /
by Gerald A. Melchiode with Bill Sloan.
p.   cm.
"An Owl book."
Includes index.
ISBN 0-8050-6060-X (pb : alk. paper)
1.   Sildenafil—Popular works.   2.   Impotence—Chemotherapy.
3.   Sex.   I. Sloan,   Bill.   II.   Title.
RC889.M379   1999   98-43122
616.6'92061—dc21   CIP

Henry Holt books are available for special promotions and
premiums. For details contact: Director, Special Markets.

First Edition 1999

Designed by Kate Nichols

Printed in the United States of America
All first editions are printed on acid-free paper. ∞

10   9   8   7   6   5   4   3   2   1

Contents

Beyond Viagra

1
Waiting for Viagra

Viagra.

Few words in medical history have entered the mainstream of our vocabulary more quickly or forcefully. To those familiar with the Latin languages, its correct pronunciation would seem to be *Vee-AH-grah,* but the manufacturer prefers to call it *Vy-AH-grah,* and the newscasters say *Vy-AG-rah,* to rhyme with "Niagara."

Regardless of how you pronounce it, though, the definition of Viagra is still the same. It's the first effective oral treatment ever discovered for male impotency and one of the most sought-after pills in the annals of pharmacology.

Amazing as it seems, just a year ago almost no one in this country had ever heard or read the word *Viagra.* Now some version of it seems to be on everybody's lips. Doctors from coast to coast have been swamped with patients clamoring for it. Within two weeks after it was introduced in drugstores, some forty thousand prescriptions a day were being written for it, a record that no previous drug had come within a mile of matching, and total 1998 sales were projected at over $1 billion. Fueling the demand were innumerable newspaper and magazine articles, radio talk shows, and TV news programs.

Viagra is literally changing our world before our very eyes—and with good reason.

True "miracle drugs" have come along only a few times in recorded history, but this little blue pill, approved by the U.S. Food and Drug Administration in late March 1998 after years of testing in America and Europe, seems to merit this definition. Viagra temporarily "cures" male impotency in the vast majority of men who take it—predictably, painlessly, in a matter of minutes, and with almost no observable side effects.

By the time it became available by prescription in April 1998, I had already had a close relationship with Viagra and its U.S. manufacturer for a number of months. As a practicing psychiatrist specializing in the treatment of male sexual disorders, I was among a select few doctors who prescribed the drug for patients prior to its general availability. I was also asked by Pfizer Inc., the giant pharmaceutical company that markets Viagra, to serve as a consultant to help familiarize the rest of the nation's medical community with the drug.

Because of this experience, I can now say that both as a pharmaceutical agent and a social trendsetter, Viagra is everything it's cracked up to be. And for better or worse, it has the potential to be much, much more.

"It really works and it takes only one pill to do the trick," says a sixty-two-year-old user who participated in a hospital-based Viagra testing program. "Within forty-five minutes, I had an erection like I haven't had since I was thirty or so—and my first one in months. It almost made me feel like a kid again."

Not even the widely hailed antidepressant Prozac has generated such overwhelming interest on the part of the public. Viagra is a cinch to become the most widely consumed prescription drug in at least three decades. It's also well on its way to becoming the most *abused* prescription drug in history. But this is only the tip of the iceberg. The real impact of Viagra goes far beyond these immediate effects. Its introduction is a cultural landmark that will, in all likelihood, alter social patterns, sexual mores, and basic human relationships for generations to come. It has already rerouted America's entire approach to male impotency—and to sex itself, for that matter. It has done so rapidly, dramatically, and probably forever.

As *Newsweek* observed some six months before the drug's release, if Viagra makes enough of the nation's thirty-eight million baby boomers feel like "virile teenagers" again, it could touch off another sexual revolution.

The prediction has proved highly accurate. This revolution could be even more far-reaching and profound than the one triggered by the appearance of the birth-control pill in the late 1960s. By the turn of the century, the drug will be available around the world, and it will be followed by other oral impotency medications.

A Long Time Coming

Civilization has waited an incredibly long time for Viagra and the other oral drugs for male impotency that are sure to follow it. By the time the first U.S. prescriptions for Viagra were written, the ailment known in medical circles as erectile dysfunction had quietly reached epidemic proportions. And despite all our other medical advances, no single treatment for impotency had yet even come close to yielding satisfying results.

Before Viagra, the only sure way for an impotent man to get and maintain an erection was with penile prostheses, vacuum pumps, hypodermic needles (ouch!), or urethral implants. They took most of the spontaneity out of the sex act, produced erections that wouldn't go away for hours (or sometimes even days), often hurt like hell, and in some instances were downright dangerous.

At best, these were ugly alternatives to a sexually lifeless existence, but they were the only "quick fixes" we had. Almost overnight, Viagra has changed all that.

It couldn't have happened at a more propitious time. There is compelling evidence that male sexual dysfunction is more widespread today than at any previous point in human history—and yet it is certainly nothing new. As far as we know, impotency has been affecting certain men since the dawn of time. Until the past few decades, however, the subject was so shrouded in secrecy and shame that medical science had developed little solid information about it.

Today, the National Institutes of Health estimate that twenty million American men suffer from it, and Pfizer sets the figure even higher—at thirty million. When partners of the dysfunctional males are included, this means that up to sixty million men and women in this country are directly victimized by this "masculine" disorder. And even this vast number may not reflect the full magnitude of the problem, since many men affected by poor sexual performance have historically been too embarrassed to seek treatment.

Definitions of Impotence

Before we go any further in discussing how to treat impotence, we need to define the term—or, more specifically, the *terms*—involved.

Impotence, impotency, and *erectile dysfunction* are basically interchangeable names for the same problem. They simply mean that, at least part of the time, a man is unable to obtain an erection sufficiently rigid for sexual intercourse. The traditional lay term for this condition is *impotence,* while medical people more frequently refer to it as *impotency.* Both terms imply a degree of permanence that could be a deterrent to effective treatment. *Erectile dysfunction* is a more recent term that may sound somewhat less ominous to the patient. It is now widely used by physicians in an effort to describe more clearly what the other terms mean.

Sexual dysfunction is a broader term that can include not only erectile failure but a variety of other problems in both men and women. (Yes, a surprising number of women suffer from sexual dysfunction, too, and many are unaware of their problems, because they are less obvious than men's. Viagra offers intriguing possibilities for helping sexually troubled women, and these are the focus of a chapter later in this book.)

Of all male sexual disorders, erectile dysfunction is by far the most common, but the degrees of dysfunction vary widely from patient to patient, and several systems have been established for differentiating among them.

The authoritative Massachusetts Male Aging Study (MMAS) used a three-tier definition to calculate how many of the study's subjects suffered some form of diagnosable erectile dysfunction:

- Minimal dysfunction meant that a man was *usually* able to get and keep an erection sufficient for sexual intercourse.
- Moderate dysfunction meant that a man could *sometimes* get and keep a good enough erection for sexual intercourse.
- Complete dysfunction was defined as meaning a man could *never* get and keep an erection sufficient for sexual intercourse.

The MMAS study also found that 52 percent of the 1,290 men, aged forty to seventy, who participated in it were affected by one of these three phases. The minimal category accounted for 17.2 percent of the men, the moderate category for 25.2 percent, and the complete category for 9.6 percent.

If these findings can be extrapolated to the general population, they mean that more than half of all men in this age group are affected by some degree of erectile dysfunction. If the old adage that "misery loves company" actually holds true, simply realizing this fact should provide some measure of reassurance for the legions of sexually impaired men in this country.

Ancient Times Versus Modern

I've seen firsthand—and tried to alleviate—the demoralizing, ego-destroying psychological impact of impotency on hundreds of male patients during the relatively enlightened era of the past thirty years. In many of them, the precise cause of the problem was elusive and difficult to pinpoint. Impotency may be purely physical in nature, or it may be totally psychological. Other times, it may be a complex combination of both.

There are many triggers for impotency, and despite all our research, there is still much to be learned about it, even today. I can only imagine the hopelessness and silent torment suffered in earlier times by men who found themselves sexually "dead," with no prospects of effective treatment, much less a cure.

It seems probable, however, that male impotency was a much less common condition in the ancient world than it is in the modern one. One reason for this is that not nearly as many men survived to reach what we now refer to as "middle age"—the over-forty period when male sexual dysfunction is most prevalent. Just a couple of hundred years ago, a man was considered "old" when he reached his fifties, an age that now falls within our definition of the "prime of life." In the mid–nineteenth century, for example, a typical man in this age group had spent decades working twelve-hour days and six-day weeks, usually at hard physical labor. Under the circumstances, he could easily blame a flagging sex drive on sheer fatigue. And the lack of effective birth-control measures often made it prudent to reduce or curtail sexual activity at that point in life, anyway.

This is in sharp contrast to our attitudes and practices today, when many men are starting second families in their fifties and when millions of men and women are obsessed with the "cult of youth," of which sex is viewed as an indispensable part. In movies, television, and every other modern entertainment and communications medium, sex and sexuality are inseparably linked with youth, glamour, and success. In this atmosphere, losing your ability to have sex can seem as crushing as losing a limb or an eye—possibly even more so.

Barry W., a fifty-seven-year-old salesman who came to me after prostate surgery left him impotent, expressed it this way: "The operation saved my life, but it also left me feeling like a big part of that life was gone forever. Sometimes it was as if I wasn't even the same person I'd been before."

Longer Life, Higher Risk

We're living far longer than our forebears. A baby boy born today has a life expectancy of about seventy-three years, and a healthy man in his mid-fifties can expect to live to eighty or beyond. That's the good news. The bad news is that as men age, their odds of developing sexual dysfunction gradually increase. Diseases such as diabetes, prostate cancer, hypertension, and atherosclerosis often trigger a loss of sexual function, and so do many of the drugs and surgical procedures used to treat these ailments. As in Barry's case, once-fatal diseases are now often held in check, and the life span is extended, but as a consequence the patient's sexuality can be damaged or obliterated completely.

Even in the absence of any disease or other identifiable cause for erectile dysfunction, the aging process itself affects sexual response. Some men in their seventies have fathered children, and some men have maintained an active sex life into their eighties. But for many others, the desire for sex fades years earlier with no identifiable physical cause.

It can be argued, however—and, in fact, has been demonstrated in studies of elderly populations—that continuing to engage in sex, even on an infrequent basis, benefits the general health of older people and is associated, in particular, with a healthy prostate in older men. Viagra clearly puts these benefits within the reach of millions of men in their sixties, seventies, eighties, and beyond, but the social consequences of so many men continuing sexual activity into old age aren't nearly so easy to predict.

Population studies show that by 2020, about 20 percent of all Americans will be over sixty-five. As the baby-boom generation of the 1940s and '50s enters middle age and the nation's population grows steadily older, more and more men will be living with degenerative-disease processes that can produce additional millions of cases of impotency. Medical authorities quoted on a recent edition of ABC's *20/20* estimate that erectile dysfunction will affect more than 50 percent of all American males between the ages of forty and seventy.

This is a stunning statistic. What it means is that once a man enters this age group, his odds of developing erectile dysfunction are at least as high as his odds of avoiding it. If this doesn't constitute an epidemic, I don't know what would.

But what it also means is that within a couple of decades, the market for Viagra and other anti-impotency and erection-enhancing drugs—just among the elderly—will be gargantuan.

Meanwhile, the very pressures and excesses of modern life also contribute immeasurably to the impotency problem. The abuse of alcohol and/or illegal drugs is frequently an underlying cause of male sexual failure, and recent studies show that men who smoke cigarettes are seven times as likely to develop erectile dysfunction as nonsmoking men. Millions of Americans of both sexes suffer from clinical depression, which robs them of their zest for life and their interest in sex. In either partner in a relationship, severe untreated depression can mean the end of sexual intimacy.

Each of these factors contributes to the prevalence of sexual dysfunction. Each represents another reason why the modern world has waited so desperately for Viagra and the "magic bullet" it represents. But the factors cited above are some of the easier ones to identify. There are other, far more complicated problems that often lie buried far beneath the surface. And instead of offering a quick, painless solution to these problems, the improper use of Viagra or other oral impotency medications could actually make them worse.

A Fly in the Ointment?

This is why, as exciting as Viagra's track record has been thus far, some sex therapists, marriage counselors, and sociologists are urging caution. They warn that widespread use of the drug could become a sort of "Trojan horse" for sexually troubled men and their mates. Without a sound system of controls, some experts fear that Viagra could end up damaging as many relationships as it benefits—conceivably even more.

The causes of psychologically induced impotence are often deep-rooted and obscure. They usually relate to much more than merely the physical act of sex itself. No pill, no matter how effective, can magically make up for the loss of romantic feeling and the erosion of affection that frequently set the stage for male impotence. It can do nothing, for example, to rekindle desire in a wife embittered by the idea that her husband is no longer physically attracted to her or angered by his refusal to admit his problem and seek treatment. (Indeed, even the promise of a "potency pill" that helped up to 92 percent of the men involved in European studies may not be enough to persuade some American males to swallow their pride—and a perceived threat to their manhood—long enough to consult a physician about their sexual difficulties.)

It's important to understand that, in the vast majority of cases, men's sexual failures don't take place in isolation. They almost always affect at least one other person. Typically, when a man begins having difficulty getting erections, his partner doesn't know the cause or how to deal with it. Her first impulse may be to blame herself for not being sexy or attractive enough anymore. Then, as the man grows more worried about his difficulty, he tends to make matters worse by avoiding intimate contact with his wife. He often withdraws from her, both physically and emotionally.

Over time, the partner's self-blame often turns to frustration. She urges the man to seek help, but the thought of telling a doctor about his problem is too humiliating for him to bear—so he does nothing. Gradually the woman's suppressed resentment and bitterness grows, while the husband tries to ignore the problem and his own nagging sense of failure and guilt. Sometimes, the relationship falls apart, but many couples reach some sort of compromise in which they continue to live together but with very little physical contact, very little affection—and no sex.

Now imagine this scenario: Suddenly, a marvelous pill comes along that promises to restore the man's sexual prowess. The man is excited and eager. All he wants is a physician willing to write a prescription for the pill. Forty-five minutes after he swallows his first one, he's raring to go. But what about his partner?

"Not so fast," his wife responds. "What about all these years I've been asking you to do something—see a doctor or a marriage counselor—and you've only buried your head deeper in the sand? What about all the times you've avoided me? Now you're all

worked up again and demanding sex, but why should I feel any affection toward you? Why should I say, 'Oh, fine, let's get it on!' and
just forget all the rest?"

The point is that even a "magic bullet" can be used to shoot
oneself in the foot. Simply taking a pill and getting an erection
isn't going to erase all the hidden scars, negative undercurrents,
and stored-up antagonisms that can mar and threaten a relationship.

The penile prostheses that some men had implanted beginning
in the 1970s produced what could be termed a perpetual erection,
and the vacuum pumps and injections that came later also made
sex a mechanical possibility. But oddly enough, many of the men
who tried these devices never employed them for sexual intercourse
with their partners. In fact, the partners were seldom even included
in the decisions to use the devices in the first place, and they were
understandably turned off by them. The devices and the kind of
sexual activity they made possible seemed too mechanical, awkward, inconvenient, and unnatural. It was devoid of the feelings of
warmth, closeness, and spontaneity that most of the men and their
partners really wanted.

To ensure that Viagra doesn't become just another turnoff for
many women, it should be used with reason and in combination
with effective counseling when needed. Unquestionably, Viagra
produces a natural-feeling erection and allows completely natural
sex. But this time medical technology mustn't overlook the importance of the partner. Indiscriminate overuse of the drug simply to
embellish a "macho stud" image could be disastrous. It could lead
to increased infidelity and promiscuity, additional weakening of the
already-beleaguered family unit, and further unraveling of our social fabric.

The Changing Female Role

Once upon a time, we lived in a world totally dominated by males.
Before the twentieth century, masculine rule of major social, political, and economic systems was virtually absolute and seldom chal-

lenged. Men made all the important decisions, and women were simply expected to follow along. As I'm sure you've noticed, times have really changed!

In the thirty or so years since the emergence of the women's movement in this country, a massive shift in the balance of power has taken place—in government, business, science, education, religion, and elsewhere. But in no area of society has the new posture and status of women been more keenly felt than in marriage, child-rearing, and other key personal relationships.

Countless women have abandoned their traditional roles as homemakers and mothers in search of equality and fulfillment. Today, they compete boldly with men in the world at large, often out-performing their male counterparts. Many women make more money than their husbands. Many hold positions as top managers and executives. They demonstrate their independence daily in hundreds of corporate boardrooms—and, perhaps even more significantly, in tens of millions of bedrooms.

It isn't the purpose of this book to debate the pros and cons of this socio-economic phenomenon. History will ultimately determine the full effect of the changing female role on Western civilization. I also don't mean to imply that it's wrong for women to take a more active, demonstrative role in sex, whether it be in letting their partners know what they like and don't like, or in helping their partners work through sexual difficulties. For every impotent man in a committed relationship, his problem is very much a woman's problem, too. But at the same time, it would be a mistake to ignore the new assertiveness of women as it relates to the current epidemic of male sexual dysfunction.

The old image of the male as the perpetual aggressor or pursuer in romantic and sexual encounters no longer holds true. Younger women, especially, have ripped up the double standard that prevailed for thousands of years and tossed it to the winds. Many of them show no more qualms than men about initiating intimacy with attractive members of the opposite sex. Whether men can admit it or not, this challenge to the traditional male role makes many of them apprehensive and uncomfortable.

On average, until the recent past, boys tended to become sexually active at an earlier age than girls, but this, too, is changing. Surveys show that nearly one in every five girls under the age of fifteen is sexually active. Girls as young as thirteen, responding to questions on one such survey, expressed the belief that "if you know a boy for a few hours and like him, it's okay to have sex with him."

While the fear of AIDS and the HIV virus has served as a strong deterrent to casual sex among more mature men and women in recent years, adolescents often seem to ignore the threat. Meanwhile, the effectiveness and availability of birth-control pills (many parents readily admit supplying the pills for their sexually active teenage daughters) have also loosened traditional sexual restraints among adolescent girls.

These factors, coupled with the rise of feminism and the demand that women enjoy the same sexual prerogatives as men, have created a whole "new morality" where casual sex is concerned. As any qualified sex therapist can tell you, aggressive sexual behavior by women triggers performance anxiety in a sizable percentage of men. This can lead directly to erectile dysfunction, particularly in men accustomed to more traditional partners and relationships. Even young, healthy males can be affected.

A "Scary" Experience

Consider the plight of Greg C., a recently divorced businessman in his early forties. Greg had been married for nearly twenty years to a shy woman with little interest in sex, but after his marriage ended, he found himself frequenting singles bars again in search of female companionship.

"I wasn't prepared at all for the way things have changed out there," Greg admitted. "To me, it was really scary."

The first time Greg found himself in an intimate situation with a younger woman he had met in a bar, it had been several months since he'd last had sex. Initially, he became strongly aroused, but when the critical moment came and his partner grew more demanding, he was totally unable to perform. To make matters worse, the woman ridiculed him, which left Greg ashamed, chagrined, and emotionally wrecked.

"These younger women can come on pretty strong," he said. "They don't like to take 'no' for an answer—and they sure don't like it when the guy they're with can't get it up!"

After several similar experiences, Greg consulted a urologist, and when tests showed no physical basis for his problem, the urologist suggested he talk to a psychiatrist.

For most healthy men of Greg's age in situations like these—at least 80 percent, based on reports so far—Viagra can provide a quick, dependable rescue. It works in about forty-five minutes and its effects last for several hours. It can be taken randomly at any time a man contemplates having sex. Side effects are mild and minimal, and most men have none at all.

Even so, some physicians may be hesitant about prescribing Viagra for men in Greg's circumstances. In my view, it isn't the physician's role to make moral judgments or try to dictate how the patient should use the drug. If the patient's problem is diagnosed as erectile dysfunction—and to me that means not being able to obtain an erection sufficient for intercourse on at least several occasions—the physician should try to help him overcome the problem. I do believe, though, that if the problem is found to be psychological, the drug therapy should be accompanied by counseling in which both partners participate. And it would be pretty unrealistic to expect one of Greg's partners—former partners, I should say—to come along with him to a psychiatrist's office.

In counseling, it was pointed out to Greg that a singles bar is one of the unlikeliest places to find a partner for a meaningful, long-term relationship and that church groups, adult education classes, volunteer organizations, professional societies, and health clubs offer better prospects.

Eventually, though, Viagra *was* prescribed for Greg, and it worked like a charm. He soon regained his confidence and found he could perform adequately without the drug, although he admitted carrying a spare pill in his pocket "just in case." Hundreds of thousands of other men with the same sort of problem will undoubtedly use Viagra with similar results within the next year.

I only wish that all instances of erectile dysfunction could be "cured" as simply as Greg's, but unfortunately, that isn't the case. For those who are less interested in the superficial thrill of casual sex than in protecting and preserving lasting, meaningful relationships, overcoming impotency can still be a lengthy, meticulous undertaking. It's also one in which the patient's partner is often as important a participant as the patient himself.

That's why I firmly believe that both Viagra and this book are every bit as much for women's benefit as they are for men's.

It's More Than a Game

Today's American society is saturated and suffused with the concept of recreational sex. Beginning in adolescence or earlier, sexual messages, stimuli, and innuendo bombard us relentlessly from every side. Free-and-easy sex is the universal theme of movies, television programs, and other media products. It has become our national pastime—a game played every day and every night by countless millions of men and women.

Viewed simplistically, Viagra's arrival only adds new excitement and more players to the game. Thanks to this pill, millions of unfortunates who were once trapped on the sidelines by sexual dysfunction can now become full, eager participants again. Not only that, but they can play longer and harder (literally) than ever before. This is why Viagra is in huge demand by men who merely want to enhance their sexual performance rather than relieve serious impotency. Although Viagra is definitely *not* an aphrodisiac, merely thinking about the drug can serve as a psychological sexual stimulant for many men.

It's easy to see why a burgeoning black market has already sprung up for Viagra and why it's likely to grow steadily more lucrative in the months ahead. Even when purchased through regular, proper channels, the drug is expensive—eight to twelve dollars per pill at retail. But sexual experimenters are often willing to pay several times that much for the chance to try Viagra. Like most other drugs available only by prescription in the United States, Viagra can be purchased over the counter in Mexico. And although stocks of the drug are currently limited, the laws of supply and demand will soon make it available in every Mexican *pharmacia* to anyone who has the money to pay for it.

"It's going to become an abused drug," said Dr. E. Douglas Whitehead, director of the Manhattan-based Association for Male Sexual Dysfunction, in an interview with the *Wall Street Journal* several months before Viagra was approved by the FDA. "People are going to get it under whatever pretenses they wish. . . . There's going to be a black market."

The temptation to regard Viagra merely as a handy new device for improving one's "score" in the game of recreational sex, and to misuse the drug for this narrow purpose, is fraught with danger—both to the individual and to American society as a whole.

The often-tragic consequences of the national sex game are graphically illustrated by the soaring numbers of divorces, single-parent families, teenage pregnancies, sexually transmitted diseases, battered spouses, sexually abused children, and sex-related violent crimes. Many observers share my concern that widespread abuse of Viagra could add immeasurably to this toll. In the hands of serial sex offenders and child molesters, for instance, it could become a national catastrophe.

The worst tragedy of all would be for this revolutionary new medicine to be treated as a "dirty joke" by a large percentage of the public. To those afflicted with it, erectile dysfunction is anything but comical. And to those who have lost the power to offer their partners the ultimate expression of intimacy and romantic love, sex is much more than just a game.

For the impotent male, attempting to overcome sexual failure can assume the dimensions of a life-and-death struggle. Judging from my years of experience, I honestly believe that no malfunction of the human apparatus—not even cancer or heart disease—can be more painful to the male ego or catastrophic to the male psyche than sexual impotence. It is, as my patient Barry W. observed, as if a vital part of you has been taken away.

Relieving this soul-wrenching condition and repairing all-important human relationships that support our whole social structure represent Viagra's noblest possible contribution. Yet some will inevitably view it as just another titillating touch of spice in the game of recreational sex; to think otherwise would be to ignore human nature.

With this in mind, both the medical profession and the general public need to recognize that even Viagra has its limitations. We must also realize that its indiscriminate overuse can have dark, destructive implications. Only by doing so can we ensure that Viagra will be a boon to humanity, rather than a curse.

Finding the Right Answers

Whether you happen to be male or female, young or old, rich or poor, straight or gay, in a committed relationship or not, this book is designed to explain what you need to know about Viagra—objectively, not as a testimonial for it or similar drugs to come. The following chapters explain what Viagra is, how it was discovered, and how it works. They reveal who should (and shouldn't) take it, what it can (and can't) do, its proven benefits, and its potential dangers. They detail its possible future applications as a sex-enhancing drug for women and a life-extending medicine for the aged. They project the future effect of the vast social changes Viagra has already put into motion.

But at the same time, the book is also intended to serve a broader, more comprehensive purpose. In addition to examining the phenomenon of Viagra, I want it to serve as a commonsense guide to human sexuality and human relationships in general. The introduction of a revolutionary oral agent for overcoming impotency offers a golden opportunity for us to drag the discussion of male—and female—sexual problems out of the shadows where it has lurked for so long. The Viagra phenomenon has created an ideal environment for shedding new light on some of the most enigmatic and misunderstood disorders known to science.

The following chapters will examine impotency and its causes in simple, straightforward language that every man and woman can understand. They will show that while certain similarities exist, no two cases of male impotency are exactly the same. Like sets of human fingerprints, each has slight, subtle variations based on the personal circumstances and deep-seated feelings and needs of the individuals involved.

My intention is to give women a broader, clearer understanding both of impotency itself and the myriad ways that men react to it. I also want to help women understand how Viagra may benefit them in the near future. In turn, I want to give men better insight into the feelings of fear, resentment, insecurity, and betrayal that male sexual dysfunction can touch off in the women it robs of affection and intimacy. And I want men to realize that even the sudden restoration of sexual performance with the help of a drug like Viagra can have a serious emotional downside for their partners. I saw real-life examples of just such a downside within the first few weeks after I began prescribing Viagra.

Finally, I want to show that, despite the eternal differences between the sexes, men and women may actually be closer together sexually than they realize, and that effective communication and mutual consideration are the most important keys to a satisfying intimate relationship.

Our challenge now is to use Viagra within this context in order to maximize its benefits and minimize its risks. Our mission is to find the right answers that have been denied us until now, while refusing to accept wrong answers, no matter how easy and enticing they may seem.

My hope is that this book will help its readers move toward these ends and toward happier, more fulfilling, more loving relationships.

Beyond the immediate phenomenon of Viagra lies a world that will be vastly and irrevocably different in its social customs, public attitudes, and sexual practices. This world can be infinitely better—or infinitely worse—than the one in which we've lived until now.

It's largely up to us to determine which way it goes.

2 What *Is* Viagra?

The most heralded drug of the decade is literally a medical accident—one that was so ineffective in the role for which it was first tested that it was almost discarded as worthless and forgotten.

In the mid-1980s, researchers in Britain began a series of clinical trials in which sildenafil citrate, a synthetic chemical compound that takes the form of a whitish powder, was given to people diagnosed with coronary heart disease. The researchers believed that sildenafil citrate's demonstrated ability as a smooth-muscle relaxer might temporarily open up constricted coronary arteries and help both in lowering blood pressure and in relieving the severe angina pains that affect many coronary patients.

The drug was a resounding failure as a heart medication, and after a few years the trials were abandoned and the remaining supplies of sildenafil citrate were collected from the participants. At that point, the drug was about to be permanently scrapped and might never have been resurrected. But then the researchers noticed a peculiar reaction among many of the male patients who had taken the drug. They didn't want to give up their leftover pills. When researchers started asking why, the truth began to come out.

What was a total washout as an angina remedy seemed to have

strange and miraculous qualities for treating erectile dysfunction. These men, mostly middle-aged or elderly patients who were suffering from a life-threatening illness, told of experiencing a dramatic sexual rejuvenation. They reported erections comparable to those of robust young men in their twenties.

The scientists conducting the studies were puzzled by all this. It seemed almost too good to be true, since finding an oral remedy for male impotence had long been one of the "holy grails of modern medicine," as ABC News later put it, and it had been the object of intensive research. It took another research project on the other side of the Atlantic—plus a stroke of pure luck—to make the scientists realize what they had inadvertently discovered.

In 1991, as the British tests of sildenafil were coming to a disappointing conclusion, Dr. Solomon Snyder, a neurobiologist at Johns Hopkins University School of Medicine in Baltimore, discovered that nitric oxide, a common and short-lived gas, transmits signals between human nerve cells. Because the gas dissipates so rapidly, however, it was difficult to pinpoint which nerve cells actually produce it.

Snyder and his colleagues searched all over the body and eventually found that nitric oxide was used primarily by nerve cells in the brain—and the penis. In 1992, they published a paper in the journal *Science,* describing tests in which the nerves in the penises of male rats were electrically stimulated to produce erections. The researchers then told how they blocked the enzyme that releases the gas, thereby preventing erections in the rats.

When Dr. Ian Osterloh, who had been in charge of the sildenafil heart-medication research in Britain, saw the article, he had been about to toss sildenafil onto the trash heap. But suddenly he realized the significance of those patients who made such dramatic sexual claims for the drug and were so determined to hang on to their supplies of it.

As the *New York Times* noted in an April 1998 article on the eve of Viagra's appearance in drugstores, "Viagra the wonder drug was born only by chance and by a coincidence of scientific discoveries."

For thirty million American men, it was hard to imagine a more fortunate coincidence. But the darker potential implications of Viagra go far beyond the men it is now rescuing from impotency.

A Simple but Expensive Pill

Simply speaking, Viagra is a blue, film-coated tablet shaped like a diamond with rounded corners. Besides sildenafil citrate, its active ingredient, each tablet contains a number of inactive ingredients with long chemical names, including microstalline cellulose, andydrous dibasic calcium phosphate, croscarmellose sodium, magnesium stearate, titanium dioxide, lactose, triacetin, and FD&C Blue No. 2.

Viagra is rapidly absorbed by the body, and within thirty minutes to two hours it reaches peak concentration in the bloodstream and is ready to work its magic. (If taken with or just after a high-fat meal, the absorption rate is considerably slower.) The effect usually lasts up to four hours, but the response is generally stronger during the first two hours.

The pills come in strengths of 25, 50, and 100 milligrams, and are now available by prescription at all pharmacies in the United States. According to Pfizer officials, the name *Viagra* was selected by computer and had been "in storage" for several years while they awaited a suitable product on which to bestow it. The word actually has no literal meaning, although it has a phonetic resemblance to *vigor* and to the Latin terms for *life* and *growth*. (Jokesters in Mexico say it combines the Spanish words *vieja* and *agradecida* for a loose translation of "the old lady is grateful.")

Initially, a physician will probably prescribe the 50-milligram version of the drug for most patients. The dosage may later be increased or decreased, depending on the type of results it produces in the individual patient. For patients over sixty-five and those with liver or kidney disease, Pfizer recommends a starting dose of 25 milligrams. The maximum dosing frequency is once a day—and at current retail prices, few men could afford to take it more often.

Just before the drug came on the market, there were widespread reports to the effect that it would cost as much as $7 per tablet. As it turned out, those estimates were actually on the conservative side. Prices undoubtedly vary slightly from one locale to another, but single 50-milligram tablets are selling for around $12 apiece— or $84 for a box of ten ($8.40 apiece)—at major retail drug chains in my area. Small independent drugstores are charging almost $100 for a ten-pill prescription.

"They're really proud of it," said one neighborhood pharmacist, apologizing for the price he had just quoted.

Clearly, the cost could be ruinous if Viagra had to be taken on a daily or regular, ongoing schedule in order to be effective. However, the drug is taken only as needed on a situational basis an hour or so before a man and his partner want to have sex. (The time required for maximum effectiveness varies from patient to patient. For some, it may be just forty-five minutes; for others, it may take an hour and a half or even longer.) If a couple makes love twice a week, ten tablets represent a five-week supply; if the frequency is once a week, then ten tablets is a ten-week supply. This translates to a weekly cost of as little as $8.40 or as much as $20 for regular users—not enough to bankrupt most people, but a price tag that certainly ranks Viagra among the most expensive drugs on the market. (Small wonder that Pfizer's stock jumped by more than one-third during the first week after FDA approval was announced and, as this was written, had approximately doubled within the past year.)

On the black market, of course, a single pill can be expected to cost up to two or three times as much as the standard retail price. It will be a matter of supply and demand, and whatever the traffic will bear.

Anatomy of an Erection

Most men are well aware of the external stimuli that typically set the stage for an erection, but very few have a clear idea of the intricate chain of physical events that have to take place within the brain, the nervous system, the circulatory system, and the male genitals in order for an erection to happen.

Without an adequate blood supply to the penis, an erection is impossible, so circulatory problems can cause or contribute to impotency. Blood reaching the penis travels through a major blood vessel called the penile artery, which branches into four smaller arteries that supply blood to different parts of the penis. The one most directly concerned with producing an erection is the cavernosal (or deep) artery, which runs through the body of the penis and carries blood to areas of spongy tissue called the corpora cavernosa.

Most of the time, the smooth muscles in the cavernosal artery are constricted, keeping blood from flowing into the corpora cavernosa, and the penis remains flaccid. But sexual stimulation triggers activity in several areas of the brain, which sends messages based on these stimuli to the spinal cord, where they are coordinated into the peripheral nervous system and transmitted to nerves in the penis. Stimulation of these penile nerves causes them to release nitric oxide, relaxing the smooth muscles and allowing blood to flow into the corpora cavernosa.

One of the things that men find hardest to understand is why, before an erection can occur, the smooth muscles in the penis have to *relax*. Even medical science had no answer for this phenomenon until the early 1980s, when the intricate chain of reactions between nerves and blood vessels that causes an erection was finally pinned down. The idea of relaxing seems paradoxical at a time when the man's pulse is likely racing—and the penis itself is taut and pulsating—but such are the mysterious workings of the human organism. Despite his excitement, the man must be relaxed, too, for an erection to take place normally.

There are several identifiable phases in the development of an erection. First is the flaccid phase, in which there is minimal arterial blood flow into the penis. Then comes the latent, or filling, phase, when blood flow increases and the penis lengthens. Third is the tumescent phase, characterized by a rapid rise in blood pressure in the corpora cavernosa, decreased inflow of blood, and further expansion of the penis. At full-erection phase, the penis reaches maximum expansion and rigidity, and valves in veins are closed so that blood can't flow out of the corpora cavernosa. (The blood pressure in the penis at this phase is about as high as or, in some cases, even higher than the arterial blood pressure in the rest of the body.) Finally, after ejaculation or the removal of sexual stimulation, the detumescent phase occurs. Smooth muscles again contract, restricting the inflow of blood through the arteries and increasing the outflow through the veins until the penis returns to its flaccid state.

Obviously, with all these interrelated processes taking place in a carefully orchestrated pattern, there are many possible physical causes of erectile dysfunction. On the other hand, such a simple distraction as a ringing telephone or an unexpected knock at the door can also prevent or sabotage an erection.

How Sildenafil Works

When so many British heart patients reported having the "time of their lives" sexually while taking sildenafil, even Pfizer officials thought at first that the whole thing must be some kind of fluke. But the vast potential promise of a "potency pill" inspired the company to launch the first of a series of double-blind, placebo-controlled studies of Viagra's effects in patients with either organic (physical) or psychogenic (originating in the mind or the emotions) erectile dysfunction.

In the process, researchers determined that the smooth-muscle-relaxing properties of sildenafil are only part of the story. The drug's most important function is that it also blocks an enzyme called PDE5, which is found mainly in the penis. This enzyme is responsible for ending an erection after sex by breaking down the nitric oxide produced during sexual stimulation. The longer nitric oxide remains present, the longer an erection lasts. Sildenafil enhances the chemical and keeps it around by holding the enzyme at bay, but at recommended doses it doesn't cause an erection unless the man who takes it is sexually stimulated.

This latter characteristic of sildenafil is especially important because it allows Viagra to work in a totally different way from penile injections, which produce an erection that remains constant for several hours, regardless of whether sexual stimulation is present or not. Instead, Viagra facilitates a wholly natural-feeling—and naturally occurring—erection on stimulation.

The studies went on for almost a decade—twenty-one of them in all. They included patients with varying degrees of erectile dysfunction that could be traced to virtually every major medical cause. One study in particular focused on patients whose impotency was the result of spinal cord injury, a condition that had long been extremely difficult to treat. An amazing 83 percent of these patients reported improved erections on Viagra, versus just 12 percent on a placebo.

Patients whose erectile dysfunction was attributed to diabetes were studied exclusively in another trial, and showed one of the smallest percentages of success in overcoming their problem. But even among these patients, 57 percent reported improved erections while taking Viagra, compared to just 10 percent who took a placebo.

Viagra was also effective in a wide range of other patients, including those with a history of coronary artery disease, hypertension, other cardiac disease, peripheral vascular disease, depression, coronary bypass, radical prostatectomy (total removal of the prostate), and transurethral resectioning (the other main type of prostate surgery). The lowest success rate was among patients who had undergone a radical prostatectomy for prostate cancer, yet even in this group an unprecedented 40 to 50 percent of the men achieved erections.

Patients in all the trials were asked to fill out a questionnaire before the studies began in which they were asked specifically about: (1) their ability to achieve erections sufficient for sexual intercourse, and (2) their ability to maintain erections after penetration. Information was also collected on other aspects of sexual function, such as orgasm, desire, satisfaction with intercourse, and overall sexual satisfaction.

During the studies, each patient was also asked to keep a daily diary in which he recorded all sexual activity and rated its success. Data from these diaries showed that Viagra improved all these aspects of sexual function: frequency, firmness, and maintenance of erections; frequency of orgasm; frequency and level of desire; frequency, satisfaction, and enjoyment of intercourse; and overall relationship satisfaction.

All told, prior to its general release, Viagra had been administered to more than 3,700 patients ranging in age from nineteen to eighty-seven. Most were tested for periods of three months to one year, but 550 patients took the drug for longer than a year. Participants were given doses of 25, 50, and 100 milligrams, and very few withdrew from the studies for any reason. In all twenty-one of the studies, Viagra produced a significant improvement compared to a placebo, and at the end of the longest-term study, 88 percent of the patients—almost nine out of ten—reported that Viagra improved their erections.

Side Effects and Precautions

No drug is totally free of undesirable side effects, but after years of testing, Viagra has been shown to have very few of these, and the most common ones are mild and easily tolerated. Most men will feel no obvious side effects whatsoever.

In the studies, the most frequently reported adverse reactions were headaches, which affected 16 percent of participants, and facial flushing, which affected 10 percent. Seven percent reported mild indigestion and 4 percent experienced some nasal congestion. Three percent or less reported urinary tract infections, abnormal vision, diarrhea, dizziness, or rash.

In fixed-dose studies, indigestion and vision abnormalities occurred more often in patients taking 100-milligram doses than in those taking lower doses. The "abnormal vision" complaints, incidentally, were mild and brief, consisting mainly of a slight distortion in color perception, particularly between shades of green and blue, increased sensitivity to light, and blurred vision.

There was not a single case of priapism, a painful continuous erection that sometimes requires surgery, in any of the studies, and to my knowledge there have been no cases reported since Viagra hit the market. (There have been a few cases of erections that lasted up to a couple of hours, but they went away by themselves without any need for medical treatment, so these weren't priapism.) This is in marked contrast to such other remedies for erectile dysfunction as penile injections and transurethral suppositories, in which priapism is relatively common. With Viagra, there was also none of the pain, bruising, or blocked ejaculation that can be caused by vacuum pumps.

In studies with healthy volunteers who took single doses of up to 800 milligrams (eight times the maximum recommended dosage), adverse reactions to Viagra were similar to those at lower doses, but the incidence rates increased.

When a new drug is fast-tracked by the FDA, as Viagra was, the full range of its potential interaction with other widely used prescription drugs and over-the-counter remedies in the general population remains undetermined. Viagra was tested by Pfizer in combination with many of the nation's most widely used medications, including antacids, aspirin, warfarin, diuretics, antidepressants, ACE inhibitors, and beta-blockers, among others, with no evidence of any harmful interaction. If there are long-term hazards associated with mixing Viagra and other drugs, it could be years before they surface. On the other hand, they could appear much sooner. At this point, no one can accurately predict when or where they might occur.

At any rate, if you are among the many middle-aged and elderly Americans taking three, four, five, or even more prescription drugs on a regular basis, it only makes sense for you to talk to your doctor before adding Viagra to this regimen. According to shocking findings published in the spring of 1998 in the *Journal of the American Medical Association,* more than one hundred thousand patients die each year in U.S. hospitals from reactions to prescription drugs, making them the sixth leading cause of death in this country. In addition, some 2.2 million others become seriously ill from taking prescription drugs. If this alarmingly high incidence of toxic reactions takes place in the closely monitored environment of American hospitals, it seems logical that many times that number may occur in situations where patients have less medical supervision.

The point is that powerful drugs, particularly when taken in combination, can pose a grave danger to a careless or uninformed consumer. Popping pills simply to "see what will happen" is never a safe practice.

There is no evidence that Viagra, taken as directed, increases the risk of cardiovascular disease, cancer, or other serious medical conditions. But since there is a degree of cardiac risk associated with sex, men with any type of cardiovascular problem should seek their doctors' guidance before taking a drug that is likely to increase their level of sexual activity.

In fact, it's critical for *anyone* who plans to use Viagra to have a medical exam beforehand. Although there is often no identifiable organic cause for male sexual dysfunction, impotency can sometimes be a symptom of a serious underlying condition, and treating the symptom without addressing the cause could be a dangerous mistake. For this reason, I've always routinely asked my male patients to be checked by a urologist before I begin counseling and treatment for sexual dysfunction. Even the availability of a "miracle drug" for impotency won't change this procedure on my part.

Who Shouldn't Take Viagra?

Despite its proven capabilities as a restorer of lost or diminished sexual function, Viagra definitely is *not* for all men.

Male heart patients who take a nitrate drug such as nitroglycerin for angina pain should steer clear of Viagra because the combination of the drugs can cause a sharp, possibly life-threatening drop in blood pressure. The following is a list of some commonly prescribed nitrates. (Note: This list is illustrative. It is not meant to be all-inclusive.)

Nitroglycerin
   Deponit (transdermal)
   Minitran
   Nitrek
   Nitro-Bid
   Nitrodisc
   Nitro-Dur
   Nitrogard
   Nitroglyn
   Nitrolingual Spray
   Nitral Ointment (Appli-Kit)
   Nitrong
   Nitro-Par
   Nitrostat
   Nitro-Time
   Transderm-Nitro
Isosorbide Mononitrate
   Imdur
   Ismo
   Monoket Tablets
Isosorbide Dinitrate
   Dilatrate-SR
   Isordil
   Sorbitrate
Erythatyl etranitrate
Pentaerythritol Tetranitrate
Sodium Nitroprusside

Substances such as amyl nitrate (poppers), which are sometimes abused, should never be combined with Viagra. Viagra is not contraindicated with nitrates found in foods.

Although no cases of priapism have been reported with Viagra, patients with such conditions as sickle-cell anemia, multiple myeloma, and leukemia, all of whom could be predisposed to priapism, are also advised to avoid Viagra. So are persons with bleeding disorders or active peptic ulcers.

One group of individuals who should never be given Viagra under any circumstances is that of men with an established record of sex offenses. All tests conducted thus far indicate that Viagra is not a sexual stimulant but merely a sexual *enabler*. But in my view, the dangers it could pose in the hands of convicted sex offenders—however remote they might be—far outweigh the benefits that such persons might derive from the drug.

Pfizer is careful to state that Viagra is not indicated for use in infants, children, or women, yet adds that studies using pregnant rats and rabbits, in which the animals received up to four times the standard human dosage of the drug, revealed no evidence of toxicity to the fetus, the newborn, or the pregnant or nursing female. No adequate studies involving pregnant women have yet been conducted.

Whether women in general can benefit, in the areas of sexual stimulation and sexual performance, from taking Viagra is unclear at this point. But Pfizer scientists have begun conducting studies with women that may provide answers in the not-too-distant future. In chapter 16 I'll discuss both the potential that some scientists see in adapting Viagra for use by women and the intriguing possibilities for more rewarding sexual experiences that might open up as a result. But until research produces more definitive information, physicians should proceed with caution in prescribing the drug for female patients.

From Good to Better?

Authoritative estimates now suggest that some degree of impotency affects as many as 650 million men worldwide and that fewer than 10 percent receive professional treatment for the problem. Yet despite this incredible statistic, much of the interest in Viagra—and much of the support for a black market in the drug—comes from men whose sexual function would be medically defined as normal but who are seeking out the drug in hopes of making it better.

Months before the drug appeared, widespread rumors and publicity implied that Viagra would give virtually any healthy man who took it better, longer-lasting erections, and millions of men with fully active sex lives have, understandably, expressed an eagerness to try it. But just as understandably, many experts are deeply concerned about the potential for abuse.

Thus far, Pfizer spokesmen have been noncommittal about Viagra's ability to enhance sexual performance in men with no diagnosable medical or psychological impairment of sexual function. They will say only that the pill has been shown to work in sexually dysfunctional men. They confirm that tests are currently being conducted on sexually healthy men, but add that no conclusions about the drug's effect on them can yet be drawn.

Most of the men I've talked to about the drug don't believe this. Dozens of male acquaintances have approached me to ask half-joking, half-serious questions about Viagra:

"Hey, I can use all the help I can get these days. How about writing me a prescription for some of that stuff?"

"Don't you have a few samples lying around that nobody would ever miss?"

"What harm could it do for me just to try it a few times?"

From everything I've learned about Viagra since I began prescribing it and monitoring its results, my feeling is that these men have good reason to be curious and eager to experience it for themselves. If it can restore dependable, satisfying sexual function to the totally impotent, there seems little doubt that it can also improve erections in normal men. In a nation constantly in quest of bigger and better sex, it's an enticing prospect—even at twelve dollars a pop.

To date, however, I've been reluctant to give in to these requests, and I've never prescribed Viagra for anyone unless I was convinced that he was having genuine difficulties with sexual performance. As impressed as I am with what the drug can do, the long-range effects of Viagra are still unknown, and I feel that caution is still the best policy.

The very volume of calls for the drug has prompted some doctors to take an expedient approach simply because they don't have time to talk to all the callers. Some urologists have ordered rubber stamps for Viagra prescriptions to keep from having to write them out in longhand. Others have authorized blanket prescriptions for all current patients who ask for the drug by phone.

I don't endorse this type of free-and-easy distribution of Viagra, and I've been considerably more conservative in writing prescriptions. Most physicians share my more cautious approach, I think, but even this brings other troubling questions to mind: Is our zealousness in trying to protect the public actually playing into the hands of the black marketers and exploiters? Are we inadvertently creating an expanding framework for abuse?

We hear similar "loaded questions" from those who argue in favor of legalizing recreational drugs, but in the case of Viagra and other oral impotency agents, I feel that health care professionals must take responsibility for answering some tough questions: If the medical community doesn't set rational limits on the use of remarkable, life-changing new drugs, who will? Few men would rate their sexual experiences as perfect, but does this mean that all the others should be taking Viagra? Everybody feels depressed now and then, but does this mean that every man, woman, and child should swallow Prozac each day? Everyone is also tense and on edge at times, but does this mean that tranquilizers should be as easy to buy as aspirin?

My answer to all these questions is a firm "no." Since we physicians have practical medical guidelines for diagnosing erectile dysfunction, we should never prescribe Viagra for any man who doesn't meet those guidelines.

Many physicians, however, are starting to embrace a philosophy of "cosmetic pharmacology," which allows them to prescribe mood-enhancing drugs for patients who are "normal" in a clinical sense but who are subject to personal or professional stresses and tensions. This is already happening with Prozac, and some believe the practice is justified because the drug makes even normal people less irritable and reduces conflicts while a person is working in a group situation.

I can see a great deal of risk in applying this philosophy to Viagra. In a physical and chemical sense, we know what the drug is and how it works, at least in the short term. But in a sociological sense, we can only guess at what it may do (and what it may become) in the future.

Meanwhile, health care professionals and society as a whole must keep struggling to find the right answers.

3
Diagnosis and Evaluation

When we consider the countless factors and forces that can impair human sexuality, it's easy to understand why so many lives are marred by erectile dysfunction and why male impotency is a unique, often baffling condition.

Thanks to the great strides in physical medicine over the past thirty or forty years, the causes of most diseases and afflictions are relatively easy to diagnose. An arteriogram can quickly pinpoint a clogged artery; a simple blood test reliably reveals HIV; a pap smear or a mammogram detects early-stage cancer, and so on. Often medical science lacks the weapons to defeat the disease, but we have little trouble recognizing the enemy.

Ferreting out the specific source of a particular case of male impotency is an entirely different story, however. Impotency has only one physiological symptom—the inability to get or maintain an erection—but dozens of physical and psychological influences can contribute to the problem. There are often no shortcuts to proper evaluation of the wide array of causes of erectile dysfunction. This is what makes impotency such a perplexing puzzle.

This same situation, of course, is also what makes Viagra such an eagerly anticipated and widely prescribed drug. Its high rate of success, speedy results, minimal side effects, and easy administration have made it the overwhelming drug of choice against impotency, regardless of how obscure or complicated the cause may be. Studies have shown that the underlying cause of erectile dysfunction usually isn't a primary consideration in the patient's first choice of treatment. What the patient wants is the least invasive form of therapy, even if the results aren't as predictable. This is why physicians across the country have been swamped with calls concerning Viagra.

Since Viagra is as noninvasive as any treatment could be, there is an understandable tendency on the part of millions of patients to think: "As long as Viagra fixes it, why worry about what made it happen in the first place?"

For many patients, this could be a dangerous attitude. Two aspirin may temporarily relieve a headache, but if the underlying cause happens to be a brain tumor, the aspirin can hardly be classified as a cure.

When the Cause Is Organic

In many respects, the principal organic causes of impotency are the most serious. Often they are major disease processes—prostate cancer, diabetes, hypertension, atherosclerosis, to name a few—that can pose a threat not only to the patient's sexual ability but to his life itself. And yet, ironically, these severe conditions are probably among the easiest causes of impotency to detect. If a man has recently had his entire prostate removed because of cancer, the likeliest reason for his erectile dysfunction seems fairly obvious. (Cancer of the prostate or even loss of the gland may not, in itself, cause impotency, but when surgeons remove the prostate, they also often take out surrounding tissue containing nerves that affect the penis.)

The problem is that other, far less apparent factors may also be playing a role in the same patient's sexual difficulties.

Many different types of organic disorders that affect blood flow or the peripheral nervous system can cause or contribute to impotency. Endocrine problems, such as diseases of the thyroid, in which the gland is either overactive or underactive, can impede erections. Symptoms of hypothyroidism (underactive thyroid) include weight gain, coarse hair, and a waxy complexion. Hyperthyroidism (overactive) can cause anxiety, weight loss, insensitivity to heat, and other symptoms. A lab test can reveal the presence of either.

A tumor of the pituitary gland can cause an overproduction of a hormone called prolactin, which can also cause erectile dysfunction. Within the past three years, I've discovered two pituitary tumors (or adenomas) in men whose only symptom was difficulty in getting erections. These cases illustrate how easy—and potentially dangerous—it can be to treat only the symptom and overlook the primary problem.

Testosterone, the male hormone produced by the testes, also must be within a normal range if a man is to have an adequate sexual response. But when prolactin levels are elevated, even giving the patient supplemental testosterone is of no help.

The most prevalent and serious endocrine disorder is diabetes, in which the body doesn't produce enough insulin. Although it can be controlled, diabetes is extremely harmful to both the blood vessels and the nerves, and it often causes severe damage to the kidneys, heart, arteries, and other organs. Diabetic men are about three times as likely to suffer from impotency as nondiabetic men, and even a prediabetic condition can cause a blockage in blood vessels that feed the small nerves of the penis.

Neurological diseases, such as multiple sclerosis, cause plaques to form in nerves that may shut down normal erections. In some urological disorders, fibrous plaques form in the penis itself, preventing it from filling with blood. In short, any major medical illness affecting the lungs, liver, kidneys, stomach, bowels, or other organs can also affect sexual function.

The Massachusetts Male Aging Study (MMAS), which began in 1987 with follow-up continuing today, showed that four of the five diagnosable conditions associated with erectile dysfunction were organic in nature. They include heart disease (39 percent); diabetes (28 percent); low levels of HDL cholesterol, the "good" cholesterol that carries dangerous lipids out of arterial tissues and back to the liver for removal from the body (16 percent); and hypertension (15 percent).

Significantly, however, the impotency-associated condition that ranked number one overall on the MMAS list was depression, a nonorganic illness that affected 59 percent of the study subjects with erectile dysfunction. This finding illustrates how intricately interrelated the causes of sexual problems often are. Depression can be a by-product of a serious physical illness; it can also be an even more critical factor in causing impotency than the physical disease itself.

Drugs—Another "Culprit"

Studies conducted over the past fifteen years have shown that the medications used to treat major disease processes can cause impotency almost as frequently as the illnesses themselves. Many commonly used prescription drugs can disrupt both male and female sexual function, reducing libido, interfering with erection and ejaculation in men, and delaying or preventing orgasm in women.

In the case of high blood pressure, for example, the medications taken to control the condition are often more to blame than the condition itself. Virtually all of the most widely used antihypertension drugs can interfere with sexual function and are among the most prominent offenders. Many contain thiazide diuretics, which drain fluids out of the body and are a frequent cause of impotence.

The antidepressant drugs that have become so widely used over the past decade or two are another major "culprit," particularly the older ones. Even such highly effective newer antidepressants as Prozac, Zoloft, and Paxil can delay orgasm and adversely alter sexual response. This is also true of certain antipsychotic drugs, which may raise serum prolactin levels and possibly interfere with other sex hormones. Their sedative effects tend to diminish libido as well. (I'll be talking more in later chapters about the challenges of treating patients with both severe psychological problems and impotency.)

According to the MMAS study, medications to control diabetes, heart disease, hypertension, and depression ranked seventh on the list of major factors associated with erectile dysfunction.

Sometimes even over-the-counter medications can contribute to sexual dysfunction. A good example of this is cimetidine, which is marketed under the brand name Tagamet. Originally available only by prescription, Tagamet is one of several powerful antacids recently approved by the FDA for over-the-counter sales and widely advertised for its effectiveness. Researchers have known since the early 1980s that Tagamet can cause erection problems, but I can only wonder how many men have taken it without realizing this.

By the same token, high doses of many widely used central nervous system depressants—both legal and illegal—can diminish desire, impair erection, and delay or inhibit ejaculation. These include sedatives, anti-anxiety drugs, alcohol, amphetamines, cocaine, marijuana, methadone, and heroin.

Drugs That Influence Sexuality

Prescription drugs, over-the-counter products, and illegal drugs that can have mild to severe sexual side effects are so common that I want to include as complete a list as possible of those known to influence human sexuality, from *The Medical Letter, Inc.,* which compiled the list. (The scientific drug names are given in alphabetical order, with trade names in parentheses, followed by the sexual problems with which they have been identified.)

Acetazolamide (Diamox): Decreased desire and potency.
Alprazolam (Xanax): Inhibition of orgasm, delayed or no ejaculation.
Amiloride (Midamor): Decreased desire, impotence.
Amiodarone (Cordarone): Decreased desire.
Amitriptyline (Elavil): Loss of desire, impotence, no ejaculation.
Amoxapine (Asendin): Loss of desire, impotence; retrograde, painful, or no ejaculation.

Amphetamines: With chronic abuse, impotence, delayed or no ejaculation, no orgasm in women.

Anticholinergics: diethylpropion (Tenuate), phendimetrazine (Plegine), phenmetrazine (Preludin), phentermine (Fastin, Ionamin): Impotence.

Barbiturates: Decreased desire, impotence.

Carbamazepine (Tegretol): Impotence.

Chlorpromazine (Thorazine): Decreased desire, impotence, no ejaculation, priapism.

Chlorthalidone (Hygroton): Decreased desire, impotence.

Cimetidine (Tagamet): Decreased desire, impotence, retarded or no ejaculation, no orgasm in women, spontaneous orgasm associated with yawning.

Clofibrate (Atromid-S): Decreased desire, impotence.

Clomipramine (Anafranil): Decreased desire, impotence, retarded or no ejaculation, no orgasm in women.

Clonidine (Catapres): Impotence, delayed or retrograde ejaculation, decreased desire.

Clozapine (Clozaril): Priapism.

Cocaine: Priapism.

Desipramine (Norpramin): Decreased desire, impotence, painful orgasm.

Dextroamphetamine (Dexedrine): Impotence, alteration in desire.

Diazepam (Valium): Decreased desire, delayed ejaculation, retarded or no orgasm in women, erection difficulties.

Digoxin (Lanoxin): Decreased desire, impotence.

Disulfiram (Antabuse): Impotence.

Doxepin (Sinequan): Decreased desire, unspecified ejaculatory problems.

Famotidine (Pepcid): Impotence.

Fenfluramine (Pondimin): Loss of desire in women on large doses, impotence or increased desire in some patients.

Fluoxetine (Prozac): No orgasm, delayed orgasm, decreased desire, ejaculation difficulties, penile anesthesia, spontaneous orgasm associated with yawning.

Fluphenazine (Prolixin): Alteration of desire, impotence, delayed ejaculation, priapism.

Gemfibrozil (Lopid): Impotence, loss of desire.

Guanadrel (Hylorel): Decreased desire, delayed or retrograde ejaculation, impotence.

Guanethidine (Ismelin): Decreased desire, impotence; delayed, retrograde, or no ejaculation.

Haloperidol (Haldol): Impotence, painful ejaculation.

Hydralazine (Apresoline): Impotence, priapism.

Imipramine (Tofranil): Decreased desire, impotence, painful or delayed ejaculation, delayed orgasm in women.

Indomethacin (Indocin): Impotence, decreased desire.

Interferon (Roferon-A, Intron-A): Decreased desire, impotence.

Ketoconazole (Nizoral): Impotence, decreased desire.

Levodopa (Dopar): Increased desire.

Lithium (Eskalith and others): Decreased desire, impotence.

Lorazepam (Ativan): Decreased desire.

Maprotiline (Ludiomil): Impotence, decreased desire.

Mesoridazine (Serentil): No ejaculation, impotence, priapism.

Methadone (Dolopine): Decreased desire, impotence, no orgasm, retarded ejaculation.

Methantheline (Banthine): Impotence.

Methotrexate (Folex): Impotence.

Methyldopa (Aldomet): Decreased desire, impotence, delayed or no ejaculation, no orgasm in women.

Metoprolol (Lopressor): Impotence.

Naltrexone (Trexan): Delayed ejaculation, decreased potency.

Naproxen (Naprosyn, Aleve): Impotence, no ejaculation.

Nortriptyline (Aventyl): Impotence, decreased desire.

Papaverine: Priapism (especially in those with neurologic disorders).

Paroxetine (Paxil): Decreased desire, delayed or no orgasm.

Perphenazine (Trilafon): Decreased or no ejaculation.

Phenelzine (Nardil): Impotence, retarded or no ejaculation, delayed or no orgasm, priapism.

Phenytoin (Dilantin): Decreased desire, impotence, priapism.

Prazosin (Minipress): Impotence, priapism.

Propantheline (Pro-Banthine): Impotence.

Propranolol (Inderal): Loss of desire, impotence.

Protriptyline (Vivactil): Loss of desire, impotence, painful ejaculation.

Ranitidine (Zantac): Impotence, loss of desire.

Reserpine: Decreased desire, impotence, decreased or no ejaculation.

Sertraline (Zoloft): Decreased desire, retarded or no orgasm.

Spironolactone (Aldactone): Decreased desire, impotence.

Sulfasalazine (Azulfidine): Impotence.

Tamoxifen (Nolvadex): Priapism.

Testosterone: Priapism.

Thiazide diuretics: Impotence.

Thioridazine (Mellaril): Impotence; retrograde, painful, or no ejaculation, priapism, no orgasm.

Thiothixene (Navane): Spontaneous ejaculation, impotence, priapism.

Tranylcypromine (Parnate): Impotence, painful or retarded ejaculation.

Trazodone (Desyrel): Priapism, clitoral priapism, increased desire, retrograde or no ejaculation, no orgasm.

Trifluoperazine (Stelazine): Painful or spontaneous ejaculation.

Alcohol and Tobacco

A repetitive theme of movies, TV, and popular fiction is that booze and sex go hand in hand. Consequently, consumption of alcohol is frequently associated in the public mind with sexual arousal. This association is justified to some extent, since small amounts of alcohol (one or two drinks) do promote relaxation and lower inhibitions, both of which can aid in stimulating sexual response. But too much alcohol has just the opposite effect. Not only is alcohol a powerful depressant, but its overuse also has a toxic effect on the nerves. Getting drunk may not kill a man's sexual desire, but it can definitely weaken or eliminate his ability to perform.

In addition, sustained alcohol abuse over a long period of time causes severe degeneration of the liver, culminating in cirrhosis. Liver damage can lead to a buildup of the female hormone estrogen in men and eventually cause atrophy of the testicles and a sharply reduced level of testosterone. When this happens, sexual desire frequently vanishes along with sexual function. Antabuse, a drug widely used to combat alcoholism, can also cause erection problems.

On the subject of destructive habits that some people consider "sexy," heavy cigarette smoking, too, can take a heavy toll on sexual performance as well as on overall health and life expectancy. Men who puff two or three packs of cigarettes daily have been shown to have a markedly higher incidence of erectile dysfunction than nonsmokers, along with much higher rates of coronary heart disease, lung cancer, and emphysema. A primary reason for this is that even while the nicotine in cigarettes is clogging major arteries, it is also constricting small blood vessels all over the body—including those serving the penis.

When a man regularly combines two or more of these drugs in his body—as countless millions of American men do—the full interactive effect on sexual function may be impossible to assess. But the odds are overwhelming that it will be magnified and intensified.

The Evaluation Process

Generally speaking, the psychological factors that adversely impact sexual performance are far more elusive and hard to pin down than those that are strictly organic in nature. But what affects the body also affects the mind—and vice versa—so it can be very difficult to draw a line between what is physiological and psychological.

Many male patients who have survived one heart attack, for example, develop a fear that the exertion and excitement associated with sexual activity may trigger a subsequent attack. In many cases this underlying fear triggers erectile dysfunction. Sometimes all it takes to restore sexual performance is an explanation that the danger of a man having another heart attack during sex with his usual partner is so low—about one in a million—as to be almost nonexistent. (Intercourse takes about as much energy as walking up two flights of stairs, so when the patient is able to do that without chest pain or other danger signals he can resume sexual activity with familiar partners. This applies to masturbation as well.) Some heart-attack patients, however, are still ill at ease, and considerably more therapy and counseling are necessary to relieve the problem.

Nearly a third of all male heart-attack survivors experience some degree of depression during and after their physical recovery, and this alone may be enough to cause impotency. For others, a shift in interpersonal relationships may be a compounding factor (see the example of George and Sarah T. in the following chapter).

Psychological factors growing out of organic disease can outlast and overshadow the physical problem that set them in motion to begin with. And regardless of whether they are related to some physical disorder or exist independently, the psychological factors in impotency must be carefully weighed in evaluating the problem and determining the most effective ways to manage it. In most individual cases of impotency, the causes are multifactorial—that is, based on multiple factors.

I often use a simple three-question test to establish whether a patient's erectile dysfunction stems from psychological or physical causes: (1) Do you have morning erections, and are they rigid enough for vaginal penetration? (2) Do you have erections when you masturbate that are sufficiently rigid for penetration? (3) Have you been able to have erections and/or intercourse with other partners besides your regular one? One or more "yes" answers to these questions is a conclusive indication that the problem is psychogenic in nature.

I like to compare sexual dysfunction to the hub in a wheel, with the potential causes of the problem fanning out from it like spokes. The causes seldom act in isolation but, rather, operate in a complementary series of effects, each influencing the other.

This is why, before beginning psychotherapy with any patient, I want to know the patient's history as fully and comprehensively as possible—medical, surgical, social, marital, and sexual. It's also why I want to make sure that any serious medical conditions that may relate to his erectile dysfunction have been found and addressed.

It's very difficult for most men to discuss sexual problems with a physician, and the affected man's partner is often the one who makes the first contact for help. To set the man at ease, it's helpful to review his sexual history in detail. I've always believed that if the patient knows what to expect and receives adequate information he will be much more relaxed and cooperative.

I want to make certain that all necessary lab tests have been performed and that I have a complete list of all the medications the patient is currently taking, including over-the-counter products. I also need to know if the patient smokes, how much he drinks, and what kinds of contraceptive measures he and his partner use (birth-control pills, mechanical devices, foams, gels, and so on). I routinely inquire about the quality of his sleep, since men with insomnia, sleep apnea, and other sleep disturbances have a higher incidence of sexual problems than men whose sleep is normal. I want to check for any hormonal imbalances that could be causing sexual difficulties.

Whenever possible, I prefer to see the couple together at the very beginning, then later individually. Since both of them share the problem, I ask them to describe their sexual difficulties in their own words and in as much detail as they can offer, and I gradually guide them from less sensitive issues to more sensitive ones. Along the way, I ask specific questions and supply information on such matters as birth-control methods, oral-genital sex, same-sex contacts, sexually transmitted diseases, and childhood sexual abuse. None of these areas are easy for patients to talk about openly, but they often hold the keys to sexual dysfunction.

When the couple merely says that they "had sex," this tells me almost nothing. I need far more specific answers: Did he have trouble getting or maintaining an erection? When did he lose it? What were they doing when he lost it? Does the time of day or sexual position make a difference in his ability to perform? What about the onset of the problem? Was it sudden or gradual? Sudden onset often points to a psychological cause, whereas gradual loss of sexual function often indicates an organic problem.

I also need to know how frequently they attempt intercourse. Often the levels of desire are different in a man and his partner. In fact, I've never encountered a couple in which the level was exactly the same. It's usually helpful to work out some compromise that can suit both their needs. Masturbation can be an acceptable outlet for the partner whose need is greater, so that all responsibility for sexual release doesn't fall on the other partner.

How Couples Miss the Point

I'm also interested in who initiates sex and how they go about it. The more dysfunctional the couple, the more garbled their communications are in this area. Frequently, one or both of them is "walking on eggshells" for fear of either causing a problem or being rejected. One of the most frequent examples of sexual miscommunication goes something like this: I ask the man how he knows when his partner wants to have intercourse, and he replies:

"When she snuggles up close to me in bed at night."

Then I ask the partner: "What does it mean to you when you snuggle up to your husband in bed at night?"

She responds: "It means I want him to hold me so I can go to sleep."

Obviously, these two people aren't operating on the same sexual wavelength.

This works the other way as well. I remember asking one woman how she knew that her husband wanted to have sex, and she told me that whenever he shaved and showered before bed, instead of first thing in the morning, she took it as a signal that he anticipated sex. But when I talked to the husband about it, he told me the real meaning behind his nighttime shaving and showering.

"It means I've got an important business meeting early the next morning," he said, "and I don't want to be late."

I've found that couples who have the best sexual relationships are able to deal with each other directly and ask questions up front when they aren't certain about something. Each partner should know—and I want to know, too, as part of my evaluation—what the other finds sexually enjoyable or unpleasant. Is one or the other inhibited in doing certain acts or asking the partner to do them? A woman may not like to stimulate her partner directly during fore-play, and this may not have made much difference early in the re-lationship, when the man was younger and had spontaneous erections. But now he may need more vigorous and prolonged di-rect stimulation to be capable of intercourse.

Sometimes inhibitions can be related to something as simple as a sensitivity to body odors. A man who confessed to me that he was sexually repulsed and deflated by his wife's "dragon breath" was able to solve the problem with a couple of sticks of breath-freshening chewing gum.

I ask the couple to describe as fully as possible the last time they attempted intercourse. The more details they can provide about the setting, the better. Where and when did it happen? Did they feel completely secure, or was there a nagging worry about the bed-room door being open and children possibly barging in? Do they use mood-enhancing props, such as candles or music? Do they think of sex as romantic fun—or just another chore at the end of a hard day?

Is the difficulty purely sexual or is the entire relationship dys-functional? I see some couples who have been having serious prob-lems for years in almost every aspect of their relationship, and for whom sex is only a small part of the trouble. I see others whose re-lationships are basically strong and sound, and for whom the sex-ual difficulty is isolated and noncharacteristic of the relationship as a whole. The latter group certainly has the best prognosis for successful treatment, but even here, it's important to find out about other sources of stress on the relationship—for instance, career conflicts, finances, aging parents, or troubled children. Any of these can sap the strength from a couple's sex life.

The history of the relationship is also important. How did the husband and wife meet? What attracted them to each other? Did they have premarital sex? Did any serious problems emerge before the marriage? If so, how were they resolved? What was the honeymoon like? Were their early years together smooth or rocky? How did they handle sex relations during and after pregnancy? How have they reacted to the aging of each other's bodies? What do they share together? Do they like to be in each other's company all the time, or do they need a degree of separateness?

It takes considerable time and thought to cover all these points, but they are all very important in establishing how the sexual problem fits within the context of the total relationship.

Cooperation or Sabotage?

After I see the couple together, I ask each of them to come in individually for further consultation, and I let them decide who should see me first.

This is an involved, time-consuming process. It's one that many patients and their partners would understandably prefer to bypass but one that I insist on completing before I consider prescribing Viagra or any other drug. In these individual sessions, I assure each person that what he or she tells me will be kept completely confidential, and I urge the person to try to think of any pertinent information that might not have been covered when I met with the couple together. Often, one or both partners are reluctant to talk about certain things in front of the other.

One of the first things I need to determine is whether the wife is genuinely interested in overcoming the patient's problem and willing to cooperate in his therapy. If, at this point, a wife admits that she really can't stand her husband and is only waiting for the kids to get out of school before she leaves him, she obviously can't be expected to offer much in the way of help. This type of person is more likely to sabotage the therapy than facilitate it.

If either partner is having an affair with a third party and refuses to give it up, I don't proceed with sex therapy. Unless both partners are committed to the relationship, it's pointless to try to treat a sexual dysfunction that relates to that relationship.

When the partner is cooperative, however, and it's clear that both parties want to work through the problem, the next goal of the individual sessions is to learn as much as possible about the sexual background of both parties, with particular emphasis on early childhood experiences. How was sex treated in their homes? Were their parents open and forthright in answering sexual questions? Were they warm and affectionate with each other? How was modesty dealt with at home? Were they permitted privacy, as in closing bathroom and bedroom doors, or did they feel intruded upon?

I always ask if any adult or older child did anything inappropriate with either partner when they were young. If the answer is "yes," I need to know what happened, how long it continued, whether the victim was threatened or bribed to keep quiet about it, whether the circumstances were ever revealed to anyone else, and whether the situation was resolved or ignored.

After the patient has had a careful medical evaluation and my initial interviews are finished, I again meet jointly with both partners to make recommendations for specific treatment. These recommendations are based on the diagnosis, the etiology (or cause) of the problem, the needs of the couple, and their capacity for putting the treatment into effect.

Phases of Dysfunction

Many intangibles can influence diagnosis and management of sexual problems. The patient's own description of his complaint is essential in defining his problem accurately as erectile dysfunction, orgasmic or ejaculatory dysfunction, or negative changes in sexual desire and response.

The physician needs specific information on the onset of the problem; the frequency, quality, and duration of erections; the presence or absence of nighttime or morning erections; and how much (if any) satisfaction the patient gains from sex. It's also important to elicit answers from the patient about his worries, fears, guilt, anger, and anxiety. Discussing these matters openly and candidly can reveal vital information about the attitudes of the patient and his partner as well as the dynamics of their relationship.

Among other things, this information can help clarify the relative severity of the patient's problem and whether it is, in fact, erectile dysfunction or one of a number of other sexual problems frequently diagnosed in men. These include hypoactive (abnormally low) sexual desire, sexual aversion disorder, premature or retarded ejaculation, painful intercourse, and others. These conditions can often be alleviated through psychotherapy, medication, or sex counseling.

As mentioned in chapter 1, the MMAS study identified three distinct phases of erectile dysfunction: minimal dysfunction, in which a man could usually get and keep an erection sufficient for sexual intercourse; moderate dysfunction, in which a man could sometimes get an erection sufficient for intercourse; and complete dysfunction, in which it was never possible for him to get an erection sufficient for intercourse.

Types of Erections

Both men and women need to realize that all erections are not the same. There are, in fact, at least three distinct types of erections, and although the end results are approximately the same, each is produced by a somewhat different process of cause and effect.

Psychogenic erections are caused primarily by stimuli received or produced by the brain. These are the type of erections related to the visual or "voyeur" aspect of male sexual response. They help explain why men have always been attracted by striptease dancers, "girlie" magazines, and erotic films. Likewise, the mere recollection of a sexual encounter that took place in the distant past can cause a psychogenic erection.

Reflexogenic erections result from direct stimulation of the penis and surrounding tissues. This kind of erection is typically brought on when the man's partner strokes or fondles his penis during foreplay or when the man himself manipulates his penis. Signals are sent from the genitals to the brain and back again in a reflexive arc.

Most normal erections that lead to sexual activity combine both psychogenic and reflexogenic stimuli, which act together to produce a synergistic effect. As erectile function diminishes with age, greater stimulation of one or both kinds may be required to produce an erection.

A third type of erection is the so-called nocturnal variety, which is often noticed when a man first wakes up in the morning, and which may actually happen at any time of the day or night during the REM (rapid eye movement) phase of sleep. These are involuntary erections and their physiology isn't completely clear, although their purpose may be to bring oxygen to tissues in the penis. Even men who have difficulty getting an erection sufficient for sexual intercourse frequently continue to have noctural erections. Their absence is a strong indication of complete and total impotency with an organic cause, although recent studies show that depression and anxiety can also affect REM erections.

A man's ability to have nocturnal erections is important enough that special testing procedures have been developed to detect them. Urologists sometimes have patients conduct a test at home, using a paper device that looks like a ring of postage stamps. This ring is placed around the penis before the patient goes to sleep and will tear along the perforations if an erection occurs. The test is quick and easy, but it isn't always reliable, because the penis may fill with blood and expand enough to tear the ring yet still not be rigid enough for sexual intercourse.

A more reliable procedure is to have the patient spend a night in a clinical sleep laboratory, where two wire bands are attached to his penis and then to a graph that measures expansion of the penis. If an erection is recorded on the graph, a bell signals a technician, who takes a Polaroid picture of the erect penis and checks it for rigidity. A night in a sleep lab can also rule out sleep disorders as a cause of the problem.

The newest innovations in medical technology are also being brought into play against sexual disorders. Doppler techniques can now be used to record penile blood pressure. Ultrasound procedures can identify the fibrous penile plaques that indicate Peyronie's disease.

Most of these technical advances weren't available thirty years ago, when I began seeing sexually dysfunctional patients, and they have been a tremendous asset in identifying the causes of sexual problems in men.

Male Sexual Response

The sexual response in men is a delicate interplay of factors; it was examined extensively and described in detail by Masters and Johnson in their works on human sexuality. For a man to have a successful normal erection, his vascular, neurological, and hormonal systems need to be functioning properly and his genital anatomy needs to be intact. His psychological "inner self" needs to be on the proper track, too, in order for everything to work smoothly. Unless the man is free of conflicts that cause tension, he may not be able to relax sufficiently.

But if the man is sexually stimulated and relaxed—and if all his interrelated systems are working properly—he will inevitably have an erection.

Male sexual response follows a regular set of phases. The first phase is called excitement, and its hallmark is an erection, which can come on in a matter of seconds following sexual stimulation. (During the sexual response, the man may notice some discharge of pre-ejaculatory fluid from the penis. This fluid may contain live sperm—a fact that many men don't realize and one which undoubtedly has led to many surprise pregnancies.)

We've already described how the dilation of blood vessels sends blood coursing through the penis and how valves in the veins close to trap it in the spongy tissue and cause an erection. The nerves that trigger this response are called autonomic nerves and are part of the involuntary nervous system, which basically means that erections are beyond a man's control. A man—especially a young one— can't prevent himself from getting an erection when he is sexually stimulated. On the other hand, if all systems aren't operating properly, he can't make an erection happen, no matter how intensely he may wish for one.

Many women fail to recognize this, and the lack of an erection can cause serious misunderstandings on the part of the partner. "If he really loved me," the woman thinks, "he could make himself have an erection. Is there someone else or does he just not find me attractive anymore?"

At this point, instead of helping the man find the cause of his problem and work through it, the partner often unwittingly makes matters worse.

Plateau and Orgasm

The next phase in male sexual response is the plateau phase, which is characterized by extreme tension in the muscles of the man's pelvis. This phase can last for a period of minutes and contains within it an important clinical signpost known as the "point of ejaculatory inevitability." This point occurs a few seconds before the man actually ejaculates, but once it is reached, ejaculation can no longer be avoided.

As with the excitement phase, the plateau phase is mediated by the parasympathetic autonomic nervous system.

The orgasm phase is characterized by muscle contractions, constriction of blood vessels, and ejaculation. The phase lasts for only a few seconds and is controlled by the sympathetic portion of the autonomic nervous system. In studies, men have reported that the intensity of their orgasms is related to the amount of fluid ejaculated.

Following the orgasm, the man goes through a resolution phase, in which the blood drains from the penis, the erection ends, and the penis returns to a flaccid state. Coinciding with this is the beginning of a refractory phase, during which no amount of sexual stimulation can produce an erection. In a healthy twenty-year-old man, the refractory phase may last as little as five or ten minutes. After that, he may become re-aroused, repeat the various phases, and go through the entire process of sexual intercourse again, although it will likely take him longer to reach an orgasm the second time around.

One of the primary effects of aging, even in men with normal sexual function, is a gradual increase in the duration of the refractory phase. After an initial orgasm, a man in his forties may not be ready to resume sexual activity for thirty minutes or an hour, and except in unusual circumstances, a man in his sixties probably won't be ready until at least the next day.

Another effect of aging is the amount of stimulation required to achieve an erection. A man of twenty may need almost none and will likely notice a very definite and strong point of ejaculatory inevitability. He also may have more difficulty controlling the timing of his ejaculation, and his ejaculation may be intensified because of its high volume of fluid.

On the other hand, a man of seventy is likely to require a great deal of direct stimulation to gain an erection, and even then his erections may not be as rigid. The point of ejaculatory inevitability is usually greatly diminished and may even be lost entirely, but the older man may have more control over when he ejaculates. The intensity of the orgasm is less pronounced in older men, but may be experienced as more prolonged. The volume of ejaculatory fluid is also less.

During the sexual response, changes also take place in other parts of the body besides the genitals. The man's blood pressure, heart rate, and respiration all increase. There is increased muscular tension in the arms and legs, along with nipple erection. Orgasm brings the circulatory and respiratory responses to a peak and may cause mild spasms of the feet and hands, a flush over the chest and neck, and perspiration.

The response follows the same course, by the way, whether the man is having intercourse or masturbating. Physiologically, the two actions are the same.

Dr. Helen Singer Kaplan, a researcher and noted sex therapist, detected another phase in the male sexual response. This "phase of desire," as Kaplan called it, precedes the excitement phase and can last from a few minutes to several hours before it gives way to actual excitement.

The desire phase occurs throughout a man's life and may be very intense in younger men but less urgent in elderly ones. Like the excitement phase, it is influenced by a host of factors, both physical and mental.

In sum, the male sexual response consists of a series of predictable stages, all pretty much beyond a man's conscious control. Each is influenced by age and overall health, and all are held in a delicate balance by physical and emotional factors. Considering everything that could go wrong, perhaps the most amazing aspect of the response is that it works the right way as often as it does.

Candidates for Viagra

Over the past few months, tens of millions of American men (and quite a few women) have asked themselves the same basic question: Can Viagra help me perform better sexually? If you're one of them, how do you determine if Viagra is right for you?

If you've suffered repeated episodes of erectile dysfunction, if you've been cleared by your doctor after a comprehensive medical evaluation, and if you aren't taking nitrate-containing medications, then you're a likely candidate for the drug. How well it works in your case will be affected by the underlying causes of your sexual problems. The results will vary markedly for patients with medical conditions such as diabetes, hypertension, atherosclerosis, spinal cord injury, or radical prostatectomy. They will generally be more favorable for persons with psychological conditions, such as performance anxiety, and against the side effects of antidepressants and mood stabilizers.

What kind of doctor should you consult first, and what should you expect from him or her?

Any physician can write a prescription for Viagra, but if you have a choice, I think your first stop should be a urologist's office. Urologists see more cases of impotency than any other type of physician. As specialists in disorders of the genito-urinary systems, they have the most experience in dealing with erectile dysfunction and in prescribing Viagra or other treatments. They do not, however, routinely have the training or experience in identifying and treating psychological factors affecting sexual performance that psychotherapists have.

If your managed-care program doesn't provide direct access to a urologist, you may first need to see a family physician or internist. Unfortunately, these doctors have very little training in diagnosing and treating sexual disorders. Before you accept a prescription for an oral impotency drug from them, you should demand a thorough vascular, endocrine, neurologic, and anatomic examination and history, including the proper lab tests.

Many patients also go to psychiatrists with sexual-dysfunction complaints. Psychiatrists are experts in treating behavioral and emotional disorders, but it is rare that they are highly trained specifically in diagnosing and treating sexual disorders. It's best for a psychiatrist to work closely with a urologist or internist in medically evaluating sexually dysfunctional patients.

Most of the sexually dysfunctional men I see have been suffering from impotency for months or even years before they find their way to me. Consequently, I think it's a small sacrifice to ask them to wait a couple of weeks for a full evaluation before I proceed with treatment. This is especially true when that treatment involves a potent new drug like Viagra, which can override serious medical or psychiatric disorders that can cause disability or even death unless identified and treated.

Most men take their sexual response and performance pretty much for granted—until something goes awry. When that happens, it can be a warning sign of a major illness, and a quick fix can leave you stuck with dire consequences.

In the next few chapters, we'll examine one by one the major factors that interfere with male sexual function and what a drug like Viagra can—and can't—do to alleviate them.

4
Digging Beneath the Surface

We sometimes try to deny it, but for most of us, the act of sex and the idea of love are inseparably blended together. Other extremely complex, emotionally charged concepts—such as jealousy and trust, respect and contempt, admiration and disillusionment, loyalty and infidelity, protectiveness and control—are also volatile elements within this mixture.

What it boils down to is that no aspect of our lives is as intricately interwoven into our self-image as our sexuality. All of us—men and women—are deeply vulnerable and highly fragile where our sexuality is concerned. This is why ferreting out the real causes of human sexual dysfunction can be such a tedious, time-consuming task. Sexual problems that stem from interpersonal relationships are among the most difficult to pin down, because they are also the most difficult to think about objectively or talk about openly.

Hidden, Festering Wounds

Because of our vulnerability, a chance cutting remark by a wife to a husband or a fleeting action by a husband toward a wife can create a painful emotional wound. Often, the offending word or deed is quickly forgotten by the person responsible. But for the offended partner, it can fester indefinitely below the surface and emerge at any time to cause problems.

The story of John and Julia is a good illustration of how this can happen—and the unhappy consequences that can result.

Julia was still in high school when she started going steady with John, a college student who was four years older than she was. Immediately after her graduation, she and John were married. A few months later, John received his bachelor's degree and took a job in the marketing division of a large corporation located halfway across the country.

John and Julia found themselves alone and far from friends and family. His job involved a lot of stress and long hours, and to add to the pressures of their situation, Julia soon discovered that she was pregnant. After the birth of their first child, there were many sleepless nights, financial crises, and disrupted plans. Instead of drawing the young couple closer together, these difficulties began pulling them apart and causing arguments. Julia often criticized John for not giving her more help with the baby and the household chores. John showed an increasing tendency toward temper fits and emotional displays, which frightened Julia and made her sulky and withdrawn.

By looking beneath the surface at John's and Julia's backgrounds and emotional profiles, we can locate some important clues to their problems and reactions. John had grown up as a rather pampered only son who generally got what he wanted and was never required to accept much responsibility. Consequently, he was ill-prepared to shoulder the multiple heavy burdens of a new career, a new wife, a new child, and a new environment. The strain was simply more than he could deal with.

Julia, on the other hand, had seldom dated anyone but John and had known few other young men. Most of her concepts of proper male behavior were drawn from her father, a stoic, retiring individual who never raised his voice or showed his anger but who radiated quiet, reassuring strength. In their outward reactions to stress, John and Julia's father were about as opposite as two people can get.

One evening John came home after working a ten-hour day, during the course of which he'd been bypassed for a promotion and yelled at by the marketing manager. Julia greeted him with a complaint about his lateness, followed by the news that the washing machine was broken and the baby had colic. John's dinner was cold; the baby was screaming in the next room; his wife and boss were both mad at him; he was overdrawn at the bank; and he had a splitting headache.

"Why can't you come home on time once in a while?" Julia demanded.

Suddenly, John felt his nerves snap. He hurled his plate into the kitchen sink and burst into tears. "You don't make any effort to understand what I go through out there every day," he cried.

Julia stared at him, and the expression on her face reflected both disbelief and disgust. She had never before seen a grown man cry. Crying would have been unthinkable for her father.

"Oh, John, why do you have to be so weak and childish?" she snapped. "Why can't you just grow up?"

The moment passed, and nothing else was ever said between them about Julia's caustic putdown. In all likelihood, she totally forgot about it within a few hours or a few days, and she never knew how painfully her remark stung or how deeply it affected her husband.

John never got over the remark, though. It smoldered like an ember in his gut, and every time he thought about it, the fire grew steadily hotter. After that fateful night, John's interest in making love with Julia steadily diminished. Many times, when he felt himself becoming aroused, her words would come back to haunt him and form a barrier between them. On several occasions, the negative feelings were so strong that John was unable to perform sexually.

These failures exacerbated the problem by making John feel even more inadequate and ineffectual. He told himself angrily that they were actually Julia's fault, not his. Desperate to reassure himself of his sexual capabilities, he began flirting with a pretty young secretary who worked in his office and seemed to admire him. They started having long, intimate lunches, then stopping for drinks after work. Before long, they ended up in bed together, and John found that he was as adept a lover as he had ever been—as long as Julia wasn't his partner.

The secretary was the first of several women with whom John became involved in full-scale extramarital affairs. In these liaisons, he always chose women whom he could dominate and impress with his strength and masculinity. But the scourge of his "weakness" continued to plague him at home, where he moved into a separate bedroom and avoided sexual contact with Julia. Three years later, when he finally told her he was filing for a divorce, the ember she had kindled inside him had become a raging inferno.

"We'll see how weak and childish I am now," he yelled as he stormed out of the house for the last time.

Do you have old emotional wounds that are still festering below the surface? Are these creating barriers between you and your partner? Verbalizing those hurts to a psychotherapist may provide effective balm for their torment and help place them in realistic perspective. But if they remain hidden and painful long enough, they may eventually erupt in the form of sexual dysfunction and severely strained relationships.

Telling your spouse calmly how you feel about a real or imagined slight may cause tensions to rise momentarily, but it's frequently better than letting your hurt and anger mount over a period of years.

Is It Mental or Physical?

For years, a heated debate has raged among medical professionals over whether the primary causes of male impotency are physical or psychological. One TV commercial for a potency product called Muse (discussed in more detail in chapter 11) states flatly that only 10 percent of male sexual dysfunction is "mental" and that the other 90 percent is physical. The message here is simple: Take our medicine and everything will be just fine again.

For the sake of millions of men and women, I wish it were that simple, but it's not. I don't think Muse could have eliminated John's and Julia's problem. For that matter, I don't think Viagra could have either, at least not by itself.

If the claims made in this TV commercial were true, then a drug with the effectiveness of Viagra might, indeed, resolve nine-tenths of the male sexual performance difficulties in this country in an hour or less. Unfortunately, the problem—like the one that wrecked John's and Julia's relationship—is often festering somewhere deep in the psyche and is much more complicated to pinpoint and relieve. My experience over the past three decades has shown conclusively that breakdowns in interpersonal relationships are a key factor in many cases of male impotence, and that psychological problems are present in the vast majority of cases. Even when physical factors are present, they are seldom the only culprits.

When a man and his partner have had a generally satisfying long-term sexual relationship but are no longer able to have mutually enjoyable sex together, the real cause usually lies buried somewhere beneath the surface. When this is the case, there is no quick fix, no "magic bullet." As effective as Viagra (or another drug) may be in removing the chief physical obstacle to the sex act, it won't solve an underlying interpersonal problem.

Putting His Heart into It

To get a better grasp of how these problems can develop, let's look at the case of George T. and his wife, Sarah.

At age sixty-one, George was the hard-driving, highly successful owner of a small corporation when he suffered a serious heart attack at his office and was rushed to the hospital. After three days in the intensive-care unit, George pulled through the crisis, then underwent balloon angioplasty to open up a partially blocked coronary artery. Fifty-eight-year-old Sarah stayed at his bedside almost constantly during his recovery and was attentive to his every need. His doctor prescribed a cholesterol-lowering medication and put him on a low-fat diet, and within a couple of weeks George was back at work and feeling fine.

"There's no reason to limit your activities," the doctor said. "From a physical standpoint, you can do anything you did before—including sex and vigorous exercise—so don't worry about it."

George felt tremendously reassured. Before his heart attack, he and Sarah had always had a good sexual relationship, and he was looking forward to resuming it.

A few nights later, he and Sarah were in bed and going through the preliminaries to sex just as they had hundreds of times before, but this time there was one critical difference. For many years, Sarah had had a habit of whispering words of passion and excitement in George's ear. But this time, as they were on the brink of intercourse, Sarah's whispered message was a fretful question:

"Are you sure you're all right, dear?"

Seconds later, George made a devastating discovery: When he reached the point where, in the past, he had always grown rigid with desire and anticipation, nothing happened. He simply couldn't get an erection, no matter how urgently he tried. In fact, the harder he worked at it, the softer he seemed to become. It was as if the rest of him had survived the heart attack, but his penis had died.

"Don't worry, sweetheart," Sarah murmured gently, stroking his forehead. "It's probably just too soon after being so sick. Don't be upset about it. It'll be okay."

Going from Bad to Worse

But it wasn't okay. Each time he and Sarah tried, the situation only seemed to get worse. Pretty soon, George could feel himself beginning to tense up whenever Sarah started acting amorous, and that only aggravated matters. Later, after he'd tried and failed again and again, he felt so inadequate and ashamed that he wanted to disappear. It didn't help that Sarah always fussed over him and tried to console him:

"Poor baby. I'm sorry."

It made him want to scream or throw something at her.

George often lay awake far into the night, worrying and wondering how this could have happened to him. What had gone wrong? Had the heart attack actually caused his impotence? Could it be the medication he was taking? Whatever it was, it was almost more than he could stand. George had always been a take-charge kind of guy, the decision maker in his household, someone his wife looked up to and asked for advice and guidance.

Now she was treating him like a sick puppy, and he hated it. Sometimes, he almost hated her.

George and Sarah were a very unhappy couple when they came to my office for the first time. George had finally confessed his problem to his cardiologist, and the cardiologist had strongly recommended psychological counseling. Six months had passed since George's heart attack, and his and Sarah's relationship was at an all-time low ebb.

"Sometimes I think it would've been better if I'd just gone ahead and died," George told me disconsolately.

After I'd talked to each of them at length, the real source of their trouble began to emerge. Its origins, as it turned out, could be traced to the early childhood of both parties.

A Painful Reversal of Roles

Sarah had been left an orphan when she was very young and had spent her formative years in a series of foster homes, living in constant, fearful anticipation of the next time she would be uprooted and moved to a strange new place. She desperately wanted security and a dependable home situation, but she'd never been able to find one until she met and married George.

To Sarah, George was more than a husband; he was a human security blanket and the parent figure she had never had. She was willingly dependent on him and glad to let him set the pace for their life together. As long as she knew that George was in control, she could feel safe and secure. She didn't mind yielding to him when it came to making major decisions that affected them both. She never fussed or nagged and almost never questioned what he did or said.

These were precisely the qualities that had attracted George to Sarah in the first place. Just as she was drawn to him as a safe harbor, George liked the fact that Sarah let him steer the ship. Her attitude made him feel strong and capable. It had been a huge asset in helping him establish and run his own business.

George, you see, had grown up in far different circumstances from Sarah. His father had been a dapper man-about-town type who traveled constantly and was seldom at home. For the most part, George had been raised by a lonely mother who smothered him with attention and a bossy old-maid aunt who lived with the family. Between these two women, who kept him under a constant microscope and fussed over every facet of his existence, George never had a moment's peace. When he was finally old enough to leave home and get away from them, it had been the happiest day of his life.

Ironically, after George's heart attack, the divergent psychological needs that had previously served to strengthen his and Sarah's relationship immediately began to undermine it.

George's life-threatening illness had left Sarah frightened and deeply shaken. The thought of what would happen to her comfortable, predictable life if she lost George scared her so badly that she assumed the same kind of hovering, overprotective attitude that his mother and aunt had shown. She questioned him every day about what he had eaten for lunch, badgered him about taking his medicine, fretted that he was working too hard, wondered aloud if he was exercising too much (or too little), and so on.

George was overwhelmed by the change in Sarah. She made him feel as though he were less of a man than he had been before. Sometimes he felt just like a helpless kid again, having his every move inspected and dissected by a nosy female.

George tried not to show his irritation because he could sense that Sarah meant well. But the longer her smothering and mothering went on, the angrier and more frustrated he became. He didn't know how to tell her to back off and give him some breathing room, so he just fumed inwardly.

When he found that he couldn't perform sexually anymore, everything rapidly went from bad to worse. Sarah grew ever more anxious and protective, and George withdrew deeper and deeper into a shell of his own anger.

We solved the dilemma by helping both George and Sarah understand how it related to their early lives. Then Sarah started acting more like her old self again, and George could see that she wasn't really a control freak like his mother and aunt had been.

Within a few weeks, George and Sarah were able to resume a reasonably active sex life without going to the extreme of using pumps or implants or drugs. In the process, they gained a better understanding of how to accommodate each other's inner feelings and deep-seated emotional needs, as well as their physical desires.

If Viagra had been available at the time, I'm fairly sure I would have prescribed it for George—in conjunction with the counseling sessions, of course, and along with a detailed explanation of how it could help remove the physical manifestation of a complex psychological impasse.

But the point is that Viagra alone could never have "cured" an underlying problem like George and Sarah's—and no one should expect it to. Only communication, understanding, and mutual consideration can accomplish that.

With Viagra alone, George could almost certainly have regained the physical ability to have sex. Yet he and Sarah might still have spent the rest of their lives locked in secret insecurity and hostility toward each other—without ever knowing why.

Young Men Aren't Immune

Millions of couples in their middle years and beyond have struggled with experiences similar to the one that almost drove George and Sarah apart. But impotence isn't confined to men in their forties, fifties, sixties, or seventies. It also affects countless younger men, often with even more demoralizing consequences.

On the surface, few people would have identified Steven R. as a victim of male sexual dysfunction. In the first place, Steven is a physician himself, a well-respected pediatrician with a flourishing practice. In the second place, he was only thirty-seven years old when impotency struck.

Steven came alone on his first visit to my office, and he was as confused and upset about his condition as any layman might have been.

"I've had some problems with premature ejaculation for several years," he confided, "but I always figured it was because my wife, Karen, and I were trying to use clumsy stuff like condoms or a diaphragm and we just weren't in sync a lot of times."

"Doesn't your wife take birth-control pills?" I asked.

He frowned. "No, she's scared of them because of the increased risk of blood clots and strokes. Karen also hates diaphragms because they're too messy, and condoms because they're too 'contrived.' " He paused to laugh bitterly. "But now she doesn't have to worry about any of those things anymore."

"What do you mean?" I said. "Why not?"

"Because I had a vasectomy a couple of months ago," Steven said. "I didn't really want to, but Karen just kept on insisting until I gave up and said okay."

Steven's remark seemed to trip a switch in my mind. It was as if a bright light had suddenly been turned on. "And it was soon after you had the surgery that the erection problems first started?" I asked.

"That's right, but as far as I know, there's no medical reason for a vasectomy to make anybody impotent."

"Well, maybe not from a physiological standpoint," I said, "but I think there could be other factors at work here. Ask Karen to come with you on your next visit, and let's see if we can't get to the bottom of this problem."

Shortcut or Short Circuit?

When I was able to talk with both Karen and Steven and get them to discuss their feelings about their overall relationship in detail, the origins of Steven's difficulties almost immediately began to come clear.

As he had observed earlier, Karen was reluctant to take "the pill" for health reasons—and probably with ample justification, since her mother had died of a stroke in her fifties. But Karen also found mechanical birth-control devices distasteful and "unromantic." They frequently turned her off to the point that she became hesitant and withdrawn just as Steven's sex drive was peaking, which helped to explain his troubles with premature ejaculation.

Karen had seen a vasectomy for Steven as a simple shortcut to a worry-free, more spontaneous sexual relationship that would be "practically perfect" in every respect. She truly believed this would strengthen their marriage and make both of them much happier and more fulfilled.

Steven, on the other hand, had a totally different slant on the situation. He believed that Karen's dislike of birth-control devices had grown into an obsession about a vasectomy. He felt that she had pressured him unmercifully to have an operation that he didn't want—"steamrollered" was the term he used—and he deeply resented it.

Steven's repressed resentment and his feeling that his ability to father children had been "sacrificed for Karen's convenience," coupled with some information from his surgeon that Steven had misinterpreted, had combined to trigger his impotence.

Only when Steven was able to talk through his anger, and when Karen was able to grasp the psychological pain of his sacrifice, were they able to re-establish a truly caring relationship. At that point, Steven began to regain his sexual function.

Again, a prescription for Viagra would probably have been in order for Steven. But although the drug most likely would have restored his ability to perform sexually and temporarily eased the sexual tensions between him and Karen, it would have done nothing to dissolve his deep feelings of bitterness and betrayal.

Chances are, George and Sarah would have stayed together even if George had never overcome his impotency, although the affection and intimacy they had once known might have been lost forever. But in the case of Steven and Karen, I think the outcome could have been far more damaging. I honestly believe that, without the understanding and renewed concern they gained through counseling, Steven and Karen's marriage would have failed.

Viagra has a remarkable ability to produce an erection in most men. But can it create trust and mutual respect? Is it an adequate substitute for the deeper feelings that we define as love? Can any drug, in itself, serve as an antidote for deceit, divorce, and empty or disrupted lives?

5 Causes with "Lives of Their Own"

Lively debate continues among physicians and other health care professionals about where and how the major causes of erectile dysfunction originate. As I've mentioned before, many experts disagree on what percentage of those causes should be classified as physical, or organic, and how many fall under the category of psychological, or functional.

Some authoritative estimates suggest that 80 or 90 percent of all cases of impotency stem from physical causes while only 10 to 20 percent are totally psychological in nature. These estimates represent a complete reversal from the prevailing belief of just ten or twelve years ago that psychological, rather than physical, causes were to blame in nine out of ten cases of impotency.

It's not my intention here to argue for or against either school of thought. What I do think, however, is that such estimates not only miss the mark but also miss the point. My experience has proved again and again that tracing the origins of impotency isn't nearly as simple or cut-and-dried as some authorities would have us believe. This is because virtually all organic disease processes have psychological implications—one of the most common of which is impaired sexual function.

Since my expertise is in the field of psychotherapy as it applies to sexual problems, rather than in urology, cardiology, oncology, or internal medicine, it isn't the aim or purpose of this book to explore every conceivable organic cause of male impotency in infinite detail. We discussed a number of the most prevalent of these causes in the chapter on diagnosis and evaluation. Men who have diabetes, high blood pressure, atherosclerosis, or prostate cancer and need more information about their effect on sexual performance should definitely talk to their regular doctors about it—and about the advisability of taking Viagra.

But I've dealt with a large number of cases that illustrate how complex and interlaced the causes of sexual dysfunction can be. They reveal clearly that impotency can develop a "life of its own," one that allows it to continue unabated even after the organic cause that triggered it is removed. Sometimes, this can work the other way as well. Sexual dysfunction that originated from a psychological cause can also take on a physical "life of its own" and become organic in nature.

This may sound confusing, but let's consider a couple of case histories that can help explain how this happens.

Saving Lives, Killing Erections

To the casual observer, Roger O. had an enviable job. As vice president of sales for a high-tech company specializing in electronic equipment for medical labs, he earned more than $85,000 a year, plus such liberal fringe benefits as stock options and a late-model company car. His work took him to some of the most interesting cities in the country and even to exotic places overseas.

But by the time he was in his late forties, a hectic travel schedule, a lack of physical activity, and sixty pounds of excess weight began taking a toll on Roger's health. He always seemed to be either dog-tired or as tense as a banjo string. His doctor discovered that both Roger's blood pressure and his cholesterol were severely elevated, and the physician prescribed medications to lower them.

The drugs did their work well, and within a few months Roger's blood pressure and cholesterol had fallen back into the normal range. But now there was another problem—one that is distressingly common in patients like Roger.

After taking the drugs for only a week or two, he started having problems getting erections. Nothing like this had ever happened to him before, and since his physician had said nothing about the possibility that the pills he was taking might affect him sexually, he was totally dumbfounded by it.

Soon he was unable to perform at all. The desire was there, the same as always. It happened like clockwork about once a week. But the ability to act on it was gone—vanished. Roger was totally impotent. He was also bewildered and frightened.

"It scared the hell out of me," he said, "and the last thing in the world I wanted was for my wife, Laura, to find out how bad it was. I was afraid she'd think I was screwing around on her or something. On Friday and Saturday nights, which had been our most frequent times for making love, I started going to bed early, pulling the covers up over my head, and pretending I was asleep when Laura came into the bedroom. Actually, I was wishing I could just disappear."

What Roger didn't know—and what his doctor should have told him up front—was that most of the widely prescribed hypertension medications in this country are simply "erection killers." They have a high success rate in lowering blood pressure, but they represent a definite trade-off: reduced risk of a heart attack or stroke in exchange for moderate to severe erectile dysfunction.

And the truth is, blood pressure pills are only one of many types of prescription medicines that have such effects. Roughly eight out of every ten prescription drugs administered in this country may be capable of causing some degree of sexual performance problems in people who take them. The drugs listed in chapter 3 are known offenders, but there are almost certainly others. And when drugs are used in combination, the odds of serious sexual failure are even higher. Almost every physician is aware of this, but in the past many justified not telling their patients about sexual side effects for fear that, if they did, the patients might stop taking the drugs that could save their lives. Judging from the "better dead than impotent" sentiments voiced by many men, the doctors may very well have been right.

I should point out that Viagra hadn't been cleared for general use at the time Roger was having his problems. Now, however, with Viagra readily available, and highly effective against drug-induced impotency, physicians should be more diligent than ever in informing patients about the sexual side effects of the drugs they prescribe. Frankly, many haven't been diligent enough in the past. They would almost certainly tell a patient if a drug could cause palpitations, stomach cramps, skin rashes, or other severe physical symptoms, yet not consider sexual dysfunction sufficiently "serious" to issue a warning.

I believe that physicians owe their patients straightforward information and that, when warranted, they should consider prescribing Viagra to offset the sexual effects of other medications. (We'll talk more about misinformation and ignorance—on the part of both physicians and patients—in chapter 6.)

A Case of Mind over Matter

When Roger went back to his doctor and told him what was happening, the physician readily admitted that the drugs were "probably" to blame. He switched Roger to another type of blood pressure medicine, but after several weeks there was no change in Roger's sexual dysfunction.

At this point, the physician suggested another possible course of action—one he had mentioned in passing several times in the past, but one that he assumed the typical patient would find difficult, if not impossible, to follow.

"As I've told you before, there are some other things you can do that might keep your blood pressure and cholesterol under control if you want to try them," the doctor said. "But they'll involve a lot more effort and dedication on your part than just swallowing a couple of pills every day. I want you to understand that it won't be a quick fix or an easy one. That's why most patients would rather take pills."

"Just tell me what it is," Roger said. "I'm willing to do anything to get my sex life back. I don't think I can stand to live like this."

The doctor put Roger on an exercise program calling for thirty to forty-five minutes of vigorous aerobic activity—such as walking, jogging, stationary running, or cycling—at least five days per week. He also put him on a strict low-fat diet, told him to cut his salt consumption to an absolute minimum, and urged him to eat a lot of fresh fruits and vegetables to increase his intake of potassium.

"Stay with this regimen for several weeks and lose at least ten pounds, then we'll see about reducing your medications," the doctor said. "If your blood pressure and cholesterol look okay in a month or so, maybe we can stop the pills for a while to see what happens."

Roger religiously pursued his new diet and exercise program. Within a couple of months, he shed more than twenty pounds. He looked and felt healthier and more energetic than he had in years, and the doctor was sufficiently impressed with Roger's blood pressure and cholesterol readings to discontinue the drugs on a trial basis.

Everything was fine, except for one problem: Roger still couldn't get an erection, and he eventually came to talk to me.

"It's really been tough, doing all this stuff," he said, "and now I just wonder if it was worth it. I mean, I know I'm in a lot better shape than I was, and that's great, but at the same time, I feel cheated. The main reason I changed my whole lifestyle was to get my love life back, but that hasn't happened, and now I'm wondering if it ever will. I get aroused, and it seems like I'm about to have an erection, but then something goes wrong."

"Have you talked to your wife about it?" I asked.

"I've tried to, but Laura's just as confused and upset as I am. She seems to think she doesn't turn me on anymore, and nothing could be further from the truth. She's just as sexy as she ever was, and I know the problem's strictly with me, but I don't know how to explain it to her."

Roger brought Laura along to his next session with me, and I was able to provide the explanation that Roger couldn't. Roger's problem, I told them, was most likely a by-product of the tensions and anxieties he had felt while the blood pressure medications were making it impossible for him to get an erection.

Although the drugs—the physical, or organic, cause of his impotency—had been removed, he was still too tense and anxious for a normal erection to occur. Roger was suffering from what psychotherapists call "performance anxiety," a far more common cause of erectile dysfunction than many health care professionals realize, and one we'll be discussing more in the chapters ahead.

In other words, Roger was trying too hard. The trouble he'd had in the past had shattered his confidence, and this was causing his subconscious to assume that he was probably going to have trouble again. Common sense told him that since the drugs were no longer a factor, everything should be all right, but his fears and worries were overriding his common sense. They wouldn't allow him to relax enough for the required process of nerve stimulation and blood vessel dilation to take its natural course.

"You're anticipating failure," I told him, "and you're getting it."

I advised Laura to start trying to help Roger relax well ahead of when they actually started to make love. I suggested a massage or back rub, maybe a warm shower together, followed by an extended period of stimulation and an unhurried approach to the sex act itself. As I explained to both of them, when Roger felt the beginnings of an erection, he had a tendency to panic and try to rush matters before it was actually time.

Without Viagra, it took a while, but Roger gradually regained all his temporarily lost sexual abilities. In fact, because of his improved physical condition, his wife found him to be an even better sexual partner than before. With Viagra, the main difference would have been that the desired results would have been achieved much more rapidly. I've yet to see a man whose impotency couldn't be corrected by Viagra if the only cause was performance anxiety.

Alcohol and Impotency

Sometimes a little alcohol can help set the stage for making love. It doesn't necessarily affect every person the same way, but in many individuals one or two drinks can create a romantic mood and produce a sense of relaxation that enhances sexual activity.

But if a man continues to drink beyond that point—particularly a mature man in his forties or fifties or older—the higher level of alcohol in his bloodstream may have exactly the opposite effect. It may make him sleepy, lethargic, or irritable, and by depressing the action of his central and peripheral nervous systems it may keep him from getting an erection sufficient for sexual intercourse.

By the time he first consulted me about his sexual problems, Blake W., a forty-five-year-old accountant, already exhibited several of the telltale outer symptoms of chronic alcoholism. His eyes were bloodshot, his face was sallow and damp with sweat, and he seemed nervous and on edge. I noticed his hands shaking a little as he dabbed with a handkerchief at the beads of perspiration on his forehead.

"I might as well tell you, I've got a lousy hangover," he began. "I tried to make love to my wife last night, just to see if maybe I could do it right for once, and I botched everything again. I got so mad and frustrated that I went back out to the den and sat there until after midnight, staring at an old movie and drinking scotch."

"How many drinks would you say you had last night?" I asked.

"God knows," he said with a shrug. "I lost count."

"I mean how many did you have *before* you tried to make love?"

Blake pondered the question for a moment, chewing his lip. "Let's see, I stopped for a couple of beers downtown. Then I had a highball before dinner and some wine with the meal. . . . I'd say probably five or six."

"Would you classify yourself as an every-night drinker?" I asked.

He shrugged again, but when he spoke his voice had a defensive tone that revealed more than the words themselves.

"Things get awfully tense in my office," he began, "and I feel like I need some booze to relax. Back several years ago, I used to be so keyed up a lot of the time I couldn't make love at all. It was hard to even get in the mood in the first place, and then, if I did, there was a good chance I couldn't do anything anyway. So I got in the habit of having a few drinks to unwind. It worked pretty well for a long time, but for most of the past year, the drinks haven't seemed to help that much."

"You're right," I said. "They're *not* helping; they're hurting. Would it be accurate to say you drink considerably more now before you try to make love than you used to?"

He frowned. "Yeah, maybe so," he admitted. "But if I had some of that new Viagra stuff, I think I'd be fine. Couldn't you just write me a prescription and let me give it a try?"

"I'm not sure the problem's that simple," I told him.

From Psychological to Physical

As it turned out, I wasn't able to comply with Blake's request for Viagra—not that day or for many days to come. Over the next few weeks, I spent several sessions with him and his wife, Alice, discussing both Blake's sexual dysfunction and the larger problem of alcohol abuse, which was endangering much more than just their love life. It was also threatening their security (Blake wasn't actually drinking on the job, but his boss had noticed his frequent hangovers and issued a stern warning) as well as undermining his overall health. I told them bluntly that it was all part of a pattern, and for Blake to overcome his sexual difficulties and other personal problems, he was going to have to deal with his alcoholism first.

His dependency on alcohol for sexual arousal and performance could be traced all the way back to his boyhood. Blake's parents had been extremely strict and "old-fashioned" in their attitudes about male-female relationships. From the time he was old enough to notice girls, they repeatedly drummed the message into his head that sex was "sinful" and that even thinking about it was "wicked." As a result, Blake was terribly inhibited as an adolescent, and he never had so much as a single date until he went away to college.

He was twenty-two before he became involved in his first serious romance, and although he and his girlfriend engaged in some heavy petting, he shied away from actual lovemaking for almost a year. Eventually, the couple did consummate their relationship, but beforehand Blake had to have a few drinks to "build up his courage" and dull his inbred inhibitions.

For a short time after his marriage to Alice, he had been able to function without alcohol, but his dependence on it soon returned. He no longer had any legitimate reason to feel that making love with her was wrong or immoral—even by his parents' narrow-minded standards—but he convinced himself that getting mildly tipsy before making love allowed him to perform better.

Basically, he'd been doing the same thing ever since, at least until recently. Drinking before sex had become a deeply ingrained behavior pattern for him. The few times he'd tried it cold sober, he'd had great difficulty getting an erection. Often, just as he was beginning to feel aroused, Blake would hear the stern voice of his mother or father lecturing him on the evils of promiscuity, and he would hit a mental roadblock.

Over time, drinking became inseparably linked in his mind with guilt-free arousal and successful sexual performance. Without the alcohol to drown them out, the condemning inner voices were simply too loud and insistent.

In its origins, Blake's problem was purely psychological and clearly "all in his head." But as he gradually began to drink more heavily, his enabling "crutch" was slowly transformed into a crippling organic disease. Like Roger O.'s impotency, Blake's erectile dysfunction had developed a life of its own. But where Roger's had gone from organic to functional, Blake's had traveled in the opposite direction, from psychological to physical.

When Therapy Masks Abuse

As much as Blake wanted a quick fix for his sexual problems, I couldn't give it to him. Instead, I had to persuade him that his real problem was alcoholism and that any treatment that merely masked this condition and allowed it to continue unchecked was the wrong approach. In all probability, that's exactly what Viagra would have done. If Blake could have easily regained his sexual function, he might have felt no need to stop abusing alcohol. At the rate he was going, Viagra could have become a one-way ticket to disaster. It could have indirectly cost him his job, his marriage, and his self-respect by allowing him to keep drinking.

In other words, the overall impact of improperly using this wonder drug could have been far more tragic than wonderful in Blake's case.

Any man who falls into the habit of imbibing heavily before attempting to have sex and has difficulty stopping after one or two drinks may be setting himself up for similar problems. My advice to any man in this situation would be (1) to steer clear of alcohol entirely for a few days to see what effect abstinence may have on your sexual performance; (2) if you find it impossible to abstain on your own, get help.

Blake might easily have found another, more lenient physician to prescribe Viagra for him without requiring him to get treatment for his alcoholism, as I did. But once Alice understood the gravity of the situation, she played a major role in convincing Blake to tackle the larger problem first. He went through a difficult couple of months, but with continuing therapy, regular attendance at AA meetings, and his wife's encouragement and support, he was finally able to control his dependency on alcohol.

Several weeks after he stopped drinking, I was able to give Blake a prescription for Viagra with a clear conscience, something I could never have brought myself to do if he had still been abusing alcohol. Just as I had expected, the drug worked to perfection from the very first try.

Today, some three months later, Blake is still alcohol-free. He looks and feels 100 percent better than he did that first day in my office. Because of the insight he's gained into the subconscious forces that set his sexual dysfunction in motion more than twenty years ago, I don't think he'll ever again need a drink as a prerequisite to sex.

I foresee a time in the near future when Blake discovers that he doesn't really need Viagra anymore, either. He may want to keep a couple of spare pills on hand just for his own peace of mind, but both the psychological and the physical causes of his impotency are now history.

How much alcohol do *you* consume in an average day or week? Many social drinkers would have a difficult time answering that question, but drinking can become such an ingrained habit that a person drinks far more than he or she realizes.

You don't have to be an out-and-out alcoholic for drinking to affect your sexual performance or general health. The American Heart Association and other health authorities advise consuming no more than two drinks per day, and I think that's a good rule of thumb. Anything beyond that can have adverse implications for all your mental and physical processes.

6 Ignorance and Misinformation

Most Americans perceive themselves as being sexually sophisticated—an idea that is reinforced daily in the popular media. But the truth is, many of the sexual messages we receive are garbled and distorted, and the information that reaches us is often less than reliable.

Sex encompasses (and, to a great extent, controls) every aspect of human life. Our very existence is the result of a sexual act. And although some would strongly disagree, it can be argued that our primary purpose on this earth is to find a sexual partner, engage in sexual intercourse, and thereby produce offspring. All the values, norms, and rituals of civilization revolve around the endless, repetitive process of mating, nest building, reproducing, and nurturing our young.

It's no wonder that we have a hard time dealing rationally or objectively with our sexuality. And the problems that we, as individuals, have are often compounded by some of our most powerful and formidable institutions. Medical science has a tendency to reduce sexuality to a purely mechanical level and miss the point that every person is a unique sexual entity. The government tries to regulate sexuality through ever more complex laws, but the rules keep changing. Religion condemns "bad sex" as mortal sin and sets unrealistic sexual standards for members of the clergy. Industry spews out a steady stream of new options for heightening sexual pleasure while avoiding the unpleasant consequences of sex. Yet despite our labyrinth of sexual laws and religious restraints, our mass of technoscientific knowledge about how sex works, and our deft ability to commercialize sexuality, it remains one of the great puzzles of human existence.

Fear of the Sexual Unknown

Despite how much we see, hear, and talk about sex, or how enlightened we think of ourselves as being on the subject, when something happens to our own sexual function and performance, our natural reaction is one of alarm and apprehension. Nothing strikes harder at the very core of a person's being and self-image than a sexual problem, especially when it's shrouded in mystery and compounded by fear.

In such circumstances, some men imagine incredibly frightening scenarios when the problem actually has nothing to do with them. I'll always remember a distraught young man who came to me several years ago in total emotional disarray.

"I'm impotent, Doctor," he said miserably. "I just know I am."

A few questions revealed that not only was the man's self-diagnosis wrong but that he didn't know the definition of impotence. He had no difficulty getting an erection. It was just that he "couldn't feel anything" during intercourse and had other odd symptoms, including a rash that he feared was some sort of venereal disease—a conclusion that his urologist's report clearly ruled out.

When I talked with the patient's wife, I soon discovered the source of his problems. Concerned about becoming pregnant, his wife was using twice the recommended dosage of a powerful spermicidal foam, and the patient was having a chemical reaction to it. The very bulk of the foam kept his sensations to a minimum, and the chemicals in the foam caused his penis to lose feeling. The burning and rash he complained about were also caused by the spermicide. When his wife stopped doubling up on the dosage, both his "impotence" and his "venereal disease" promptly vanished.

I only wish all cases of sexual dysfunction were that easily remedied, but my experience with this patient made me realize how important it is to check on what method of contraception a couple is using.

It's also worth pointing out that a "potency pill" would have been no help in relieving this man's problems.

Doctors Are Guilty, Too

It's often understandable when a frightened, confused, or inexperienced patient makes a mistake or jumps to a false conclusion. But physicians and other health care professionals are sometimes just as guilty of perpetuating ignorance as the people who come to them for help, and I find this harder to excuse or justify.

Some doctors contribute to misconceptions by dispensing information that is either misleading or blatantly false, and the effect on their patients is infinitely worse than if the misinformation had come from a less august, less authoritative source. I think the vast majority of physicians are genuinely interested in their patients and in helping them overcome whatever problems they may have. Since most physicians are also extremely rushed and have only a few minutes to spend with each patient, they obviously don't want to waste valuable time on petty, unimportant matters. But their manner can come across as condescending, paternalistic, or even arrogant at times. In countless instances, a doctor may shrug off or brush aside some of a patient's deepest, most serious concerns without even being aware of it.

I never think about how much anguish can result from a chance remark by a physician's "voice of authority" without remembering the case of Warren G., a banking executive in his early seventies, who was both hurt and angry when he came to me several years ago.

Warren had developed a troubling erectile problem after undergoing a transurethral prostatectomy. This is a routine surgical procedure for benign enlargement of the prostate gland, a condition that affects millions of older men and causes a frequent need to urinate and an inability to pass more than a small amount of urine at a time. The procedure involves going into the prostate through the urethra and "reaming out" the area where the prostate has overgrown and pinched off the urethra, blocking the normal flow of urine.

Warren's urologist had told him there was no physical reason for the surgery to cause erectile dysfunction. But it was an offhand remark by the doctor a few moments later that really upset Warren.

"He asked me how old I was," Warren said, "and I told him, 'Seventy-one, why?' He looked me straight in the eye and said, 'Well, at your age, you shouldn't be worrying about sex, anyway.' "

I could see Warren's jaw working and his eyes blazing as he recounted the conversation. "I was grateful to the doctor for getting me so I could pee again, but that really upset me," he fumed. "My wife and I have always had a very enjoyable sex life, and neither one of us thinks we're too old to keep enjoying it."

"I can't blame you for being upset," I said. "It was an insensitive remark, to say the least, but it reflects a widespread lack of understanding, even in the medical community, about older people and sex. Some people lose interest in sex as they get older, but as long as the desire's there, there's no reason they have to quit at any given age. In most cases, people can keep having sex as long as they live."

"Well, I can tell you for sure I haven't lost interest, and Fran, my wife, will vouch for that," Warren said. "But I'm afraid I'm getting impotent. I can't seem to keep an erection long enough to make love anymore."

"What happens?"

"Fran and I usually spend some time playing around, you know, even after I feel like I'm raring to go. I get really aroused, but then, before I can do anything, I just . . . I just lose it, that's all. I go all limp, and there's no way I can get it up again. Isn't that what it means to be impotent?"

"No," I said. "You're definitely not impotent, so just get that idea out of your mind. Your problem's something else, and I'm sure it's fixable."

"Even in an old goat like me?" he asked uncertainly.

"Yes," I assured him. "Trust me."

Warren cheered up immediately, and the longer we talked, the clearer it became what the source of his difficulty actually was. One of the most common sexual changes that takes place as a man ages is a gradually increasing refractory period—the time it takes him to get another erection after an initial sexual episode.

Even people who know what the term *refractory period* means commonly assume that it begins only with orgasm and ejaculation, but that isn't always true. It can also happen after an erection is maintained over a lengthy period of time, even if the man doesn't have an orgasm or ejaculate. This is especially true in older men, who are usually more capable of controlling or delaying an orgasm than younger men.

What was happening in Warren's case was that he and Fran were enjoying their preliminary love play so much that they were simply taking too long to begin actual intercourse. Warren's sustained erection was ending in a refractory period before they got to the "main event." (I'll discuss sex and the aging process more fully in a later chapter.)

The proper professional approach here was to explain to Warren that, yes, there are certain differences in sexual behavior that come with advancing age, and that a man in his seventies often needs to adjust his lovemaking to conform to these changes. But it was definitely thoughtless and uncalled-for of Warren's urologist to imply that he was too old even to be concerned about sex.

Spreading the (False) Word

When a drug with the instant popularity, far-reaching social implications, and pure sex appeal of Viagra hits the market, it becomes a natural target for the humorists and jokesters. From the guys hanging around the water cooler at the office to the late-night comics on network TV and the nation's top syndicated columnists and cartoonists, everybody seems to have a favorite gag about it.

"It is a sign of the times that the only thing American men are more obsessed with than Viagra is why they didn't buy stock in Viagra," writes Maureen Dowd in the *New York Times.* "We are moments away from Viagra juice bars in Brentwood, skim decaf Viagraccino in Seattle and Viagraburgers at the White House."

An editorial cartoon in the Jackson, Mississippi, *Clarion-Ledger* shows two clandestine Republican elephants tossing a crate of Viagra from a car at the gate of the White House. A tag on the crate reads "To Bill," and the caption says: "How This Whole Mess Began," referring to the allegations of sexual misconduct against President Clinton. (One guest on a New York radio talk show suggested this little rhyme as an advertising jingle for Viagra: "Take the pill and be like Bill.")

In the *Dallas Morning News,* another cartoon shows an elderly couple sitting on the front porch on a warm afternoon. The man is fanning himself vigorously and doesn't notice his wife surreptitiously pushing a bottle of Viagra toward him with her cane. "Think it'll get any HOTTER today, Ma?" the man is asking.

In yet another cartoon, in the *New Yorker,* a man sits ruefully at the wheel of an expensive automobile he has just bought, asking someone over a cellular phone: "You think I would have sunk forty thousand clams into this lemon if I had known they were coming out with a nine-dollar boner pill?"

And *Times* columnist Dowd quips: "An unscientific poll of my girlfriends found that they would rather have a pill that could change a man's personality an hour *after* sex."

I can appreciate this humor as well as most people—maybe even better because I'm so close to the subject. And I've got no problem with people telling Viagra jokes—or with people laughing at those jokes. Some of the jokes and cartoons are hilarious. At the same time, however, much of this humor tends to trivialize, oversimplify, and even distort what Viagra is all about. In subtle, unintentional ways, some of it also spreads false ideas, serious misconceptions, and totally groundless myths. Each of the gag lines above conveys a somewhat inaccurate conception of the purposes for which Viagra is intended. Taken in the spirit of fun, they cause no real harm, but they may help perpetuate a message of confusion and wrong ideas.

Far less forgivable than the jokes distorting Viagra's powers and purpose, however, are sensationalized falsehoods that are sometimes presented as "truth." A flagrant example of this was an article in the May 26, 1998, edition of the *National Enquirer.*

The headline proclaimed that Viagra had turned controversial talk show host Jerry Springer into a "sex addict" and that the "love pill" had wrecked his life. It went downhill from there. The headline above the article on page 9 was a repeat of the one on the cover, except that it used the term "sex fiend" instead of "sex addict." The article itself referred to Springer, the controversial talk show host, as a titan of trash TV and opened with a quote, allegedly from Springer, blaming Viagra for the misadventure.

An unnamed friend, the only source for the article's claims that Springer used Viagra, also reported that Springer had loved the drug and claimed it increased his potency enormously.

The article was an apparent follow-up to a report in the steamy British weekly, *News of the World,* which claimed that Springer had been caught in a compromising situation in a Chicago hotel room with an X-rated porno movie star and her stepmother. The British newspaper reported that Springer had sex with the women, but made no mention of Viagra. After his encounter was made public, however, according to the *Enquirer,* Springer cursed Viagra, saying it caused him to lose his mind and gave him an insatiable sex drive.

The whole premise of the story is, of course, absurd. Viagra has no effect on character, personality, intelligence, sanity, or moral judgment. It isn't an aphrodisiac, and it doesn't cause sexual arousal. With sexual stimulation, it does produce erections in most men, but that's all. What a man does with his erection after that is between him, his partner, and his conscience.

But several million readers of this article came away with just the opposite impression.

Some Hopeful Signs

On the other hand, a few of the jokes and stories that have swept the country not only capture the true essence of the Viagra phenomenon but may even serve as a valuable warning to some men who try to abuse it.

I especially like the one that goes: "Old So-and-so's been staying out of bars and sticking pretty close to home lately—ever since his wife started counting his Viagra pills."

I like this one-liner because it has a moral and contains a strong element of truth. Men who are tempted to use Viagra to cheat on their partners should beware of its message.

I've overheard an endless string of misinformed remarks about Viagra—not jokes in this case but supposedly serious comments—during the past few months. A few, made by people I considered to be reasonably intelligent and well informed, were so far off base that I felt a need to interrupt and correct them on the spot. The following tidbits are among the ones I remember most distinctly:

"I can't afford that stuff. They say you've got to take it every day for it to do any good."

"I read someplace that you can go for five hours nonstop on just one little pill."

"I know a guy who tried it, and he claimed he got an erection that lasted all night and into the next day."

"You better keep your pills away from your wife. I hear they turn some women into nymphomaniacs."

More open, uninhibited discussion of Viagra and the whole topic of erectile dysfunction can help dispel ridiculous ideas like these, and this is one aspect of the Viagra Revolution that I feel could be especially valuable. The appearance of this wonder drug and the rash of publicity surrounding it have caused many men with sexual problems to realize for the first time that they aren't alone, that they have tens of millions of other men for company. Never in my career have I heard so many guys talking so frankly about their interest in improving their sexual performance and sharing so many of their individual concerns about sex as I have in the past few months. Problems that were once held in deepest secrecy are being dragged out into the daylight.

I see this healthy dialogue as a very positive, encouraging sign, and I hope it continues. While none of us, as sexual creatures, can divorce ourselves emotionally from the subject of sex, the more honest and receptive we can be about it, the better. This is probably the best antidote yet for the poison of ignorance and misinformation.

Where Medical Schools Fail

But in the long term, the only real cure is education, both for the general public and for the nation's health care professionals. Every physician should be able to offer sound, reliable information and guidance for patients with sexual concerns. At the moment, however, most doctors receive no training in these problems and lack the necessary basic knowledge even to recognize them, much less to determine their causes.

Frankly, I'm not optimistic about what the medical schools are doing in the realm of sex education for physicians. During the 1960s, we made the troubling discovery that doctors in general really didn't know any more about human sexuality than other individuals with comparable education levels in nonmedical fields, and steps were taken to address the problem.

In the 1970s, in an effort to upgrade the level of sexual knowledge among their graduates, many medical schools added courses to their curricula on the medical aspects of sexuality. During this period, I coordinated a medical school course that was mandatory for all second-year students. I also received a grant from the National Institute of Mental Health to teach this subject to residents in family medicine, urology, and obstetrics and gynecology. At the time, I thought we were on the right track, but for reasons that are hard to understand, these courses have now vanished from the scene. If any med school instruction at all is offered today in human sexuality, it's usually tossed in as a sort of afterthought in courses on psychiatry, endocrinology, OB-GYN, physiology, or urology.

It would be extremely unusual today for a medical student to be supervised in taking a patient's sexual history. I've been told by busy house staff members at a major public hospital that family medicine and OB-GYN residents don't routinely look for sexual problems in their patients because they have neither the time nor the knowledge to address such problems if they were to be found. Yet physicians and members of the clergy are the ones to whom Americans most often turn for help with their sexual problems. Except for a handful of ministers with specialized training and expertise in social work and family counseling, the clergy can be assumed to be even less knowledgeable in this field than physicians. The whole situation makes me uneasy.

Today's managed-care health programs dictate that doctors spend less and less time with individual patients. The typical family-practice physician allots an average of just seven minutes or less to consultation with each patient. This leaves no time to do anything except deal with the immediate problem at hand. Asking the patient questions or giving him information on general health concerns—sexual or otherwise—is virtually impossible. In fact, many physicians have adopted the practice of hiring paraprofessionals to handle the bulk of one-on-one consultation with patients.

In this setting, it's highly unlikely that any doctor will spend the necessary time to follow up with their patients on a noncrucial sexual question or complaint—much less to educate those patients in how to deal with sexual problems. Yet these are the same doctors who will be writing millions of prescriptions for Viagra in the months to come.

"The level of naïveté about Viagra—in both physicians and the public—is astounding," says Dr. Marty Klein, a sex therapist and the author of the book *Ask Me Anything*.

I couldn't agree more; but naïveté, ignorance, and misinformation aren't confined to a single drug or class of drugs. They extend to the entire subject of sexuality, and this is a shame—a very dangerous shame. Sex and sexual concerns are too fundamentally important to all of us to be left behind in the "dark ages" as we plunge into a new millennium.

If Viagra can help change this situation by making physicians more knowledgeable about human sexuality in general and about male sexual dysfunction in particular, that may be its most momentous contribution to the nation's health.

7 Situational Factors

Most of us are aware that sexual experiences often seem better in certain circumstances than they do in others. Time and place can be very important. We may never consciously try to analyze the factors responsible for this distinction, but we recognize that it does exist.

For a young married couple with children, a quiet Saturday evening when the kids are staying overnight at Grandma's and the day-to-day pressures are temporarily forgotten would appear to offer the ideal circumstances for intimacy. Yet, conversely, the same couple may find a few stolen moments of predawn lovemaking before work on a hectic Monday morning to be even more exciting and fulfilling.

In the same vein, we may be more comfortable about having sex in a familiar, predictable environment, yet discover heightened sexual thrills by making love in strange, romantic new places—feelings that undoubtedly influence the vacation choices of millions of couples each year.

Many couples with mutually satisfying sexual relationships schedule sex at times when they expect to be more relaxed and less likely to be interrupted. Others prefer a less structured, more spontaneous type of sexual expression. But regardless of the approach, circumstances and priorities have a way of changing as years go by, and what once seemed a near-perfect time for sexual activity may gradually become a bad time—or even an impossible time.

Martin and Betty L. learned about this kind of change the hard way. During more than twenty-five years of marriage, Friday nights had always been their "special time." They would share an intimate dinner, have a drink or two, spend an hour or so sitting next to each other on the couch in the den, listening to music or watching TV, and conclude the evening with a half hour of what they both described as "great sex." It was a deeply satisfying way to end the workweek and start the weekend.

The Price of Exhaustion

But during those twenty-five years, Martin had gone from being a young social studies teacher who left school promptly when the final bell rang at 3:45 P.M. to being a middle-aged assistant principal at a large suburban high school. His heavy load of responsibilities and paperwork often kept him in his office until 5:30 or later. Fridays were especially long, busy days, and he was usually dead on his feet when he got home.

On some Friday nights, Martin fell asleep on the couch within a few minutes after finishing dinner, and even when he managed to stay awake until bedtime, he was groggy, irritable, and in no condition for making love. When he first consulted me, he had been plagued by increasingly severe erectile dysfunction for seven or eight months. A physical exam turned up no organic cause, and after hearing all the hoopla about Viagra, Martin saw it as the salvation for his marriage.

"Betty's got this silly idea that she's the cause of all this," he said disgustedly. "She's worried about me thinking she's not attractive anymore, but that's not true. She even asked me straight out a couple of times if I was having an affair with some young teacher, and that's not true, either. I love Betty as much as ever, and she's a wonderful sex partner, but I just have one helluva time getting an erection, and it's gotten to the point that I actually dread Friday nights."

Sometimes, the people who are most directly affected by this kind of situation are the least able to see a potentially easy solution, but I had a feeling that Martin's problem wasn't all that complicated. In all likelihood, he was just too tired for sex at the end of a long, draining week at school, and I explained that exhaustion can have serious adverse effects on both sexual desire and the ability to perform. I suspected that this had touched off the problem in the first place and that increasing performance anxiety had then complicated it.

"I'm considering prescribing Viagra for you," I said, "but the first thing I'd recommend—even before you take the drug—is that you change your schedule. Explain the reasons for the change to your wife, then forget about trying to play Romeo on Friday nights. Just go to bed early and get a good night's sleep. By later in the weekend—say, Saturday night or even Sunday morning—you'll be more rested and refreshed, and that could make a big difference."

Martin shook his head. "It seems silly, but the Friday night thing's gotten to be such an ingrained part of our routine over so many years that I never even thought of that," he said. "Do you really think it could be something that simple?"

"Definitely," I said. "Let's give it a try and see what happens. But however your rescheduling works out, just relax when the time comes and don't worry about it."

"I'm feeling more upbeat already," he said.

"That's good," I told him, "but there's something else I think you should keep in mind. You need to look for ways to take it a little easier at work. Getting stressed out and exhausted every week can lead to some very dangerous health problems, and the older you get, the bigger the risk becomes."

Betty came along with Martin on his next visit to my office, and I could tell by the way they were holding hands and grinning at each other that the romance was back in their relationship.

A "Stud"—Even Without Viagra

"I'm so glad you told Martin what you did," Betty said. "He was afraid I'd get my feelings hurt if he wanted to change 'our time' to another night, but everything worked out fine."

She smiled at her husband, then turned to me and added in a more serious tone: "But the most important thing is that what you said made me realize how terribly Martin's job was wearing him out, and I talked him into cutting back on his hours and slowing down a little."

"She made me promise to get away from the school by no later than five o'clock," Martin said, "and just shaving that extra thirty to forty-five minutes off the end of the day has made a big difference."

Betty laughed. "As a result, I think I've rediscovered the twenty-five-year-old stud I married," she said.

"I really don't think I'm going to need Viagra after all," Martin told me with a wide smile.

To me, there's a valuable lesson to be learned in Martin's and Betty's experience. If he had simply swallowed Viagra, as he had wanted to do when he first came to me, I have little doubt that it would have restored his sexual prowess sufficiently to have intercourse, even in his exhausted state. But this would have been a "quick fix" that did nothing to address the true underlying cause of Martin's problem.

By taking a somewhat less convenient, less instantly gratifying approach to treatment, we were able to enlist Betty's help in eliminating that cause instead of dealing only with the surface symptoms. As a result, Martin made some vital changes in his lifestyle that promise to protect his overall health in the future.

If his erectile problems had continued after these steps were taken because of anxiety, then it might have been appropriate to send Viagra to the rescue. But even then, the mere reversal of symptoms can't be considered a full cure. There's much more to sexuality than just the hooking up of the plumbing. What a couple is doing sexually is integrated into the rest of their relationship. If that relationship is mature and based on mutual concern and esteem, whatever disturbs or injures one partner does the same to the other.

The key point here is this: If we had taken the easy way out, a highly effective drug might well have masked the extent of Martin's exhaustion, even though it got the plumbing hooked back up again. And if the stress and long hours had continued, they could have greatly increased his risk of developing hypertension, coronary heart disease, or other chronic life-threatening conditions.

As it was, Martin accomplished something even more important than regaining "stud status" in the eyes of his wife. He also took measures designed to add significantly to the length and quality of his life—and Betty's, too.

Could you be experiencing problems similar to theirs? To evaluate your own situation, ask yourself the following questions: Am I subject to stressful factors that could adversely affect a sexual relationship, such as job or child-raising pressures, financial worries, or conflicts with parents or in-laws? Could my partner and I schedule our sexual activity at a more advantageous time?

Objective answers to these questions could provide important clues for a simple solution to the problem. Remember, taking a pill to alleviate a sexual symptom does nothing to provide meaningful answers to these questions.

Being in the Wrong Place

Timing is only one of the situational factors that can bring anxiety into play and affect sexual performance. Another is location. In the familiar confines of his own bedroom, a man may have no performance problems at all, yet he may become totally dysfunctional in a place that feels alien or "wrong" to him.

This was precisely what happened to Larry H. whenever he and his wife, Alisha, went to visit his in-laws. Larry, the sales manager for an auto supply store, was just twenty-eight the first time he encountered erectile problems. Ordinarily, he was as virile and sexually active as any normal man his age, and, in fact, he and Alisha averaged having sex about five times a week, which is above average, even for young couples.

Larry had never experienced a moment's difficulty in getting or keeping an erection until one weekend about six months after he and Alisha were married, when they spent a couple of days at the home of Alisha's parents. It was Larry's first time staying in the same house with his in-laws overnight, and he didn't give the idea much thought until his father-in-law was helping them carry their bags in from the car.

"This is my old room, honey—our room now," Alisha whispered excitedly after her dad had left them alone in the upstairs bedroom. "Won't it be fun to make love in here?"

"Oh, sure, I guess so," Larry said, feeling a little uneasy all of a sudden. "Uh, where's your mom and dad's room?"

Alisha giggled. "Right next door," she said, indicating the wall behind the headboard of the bed. "But don't worry, they won't bother us."

Larry did worry about it, though. When he and Alisha were alone in their small love nest in the city, they had a total sense of sexual freedom. They could do anything they wanted together, at any hour of the day or night, and in any spot in the house, even on top of the kitchen table if they felt like it. But the idea of making love here—in this large, strange house inhabited by people he didn't know very well, and with his wife's parents just a few feet away—made him nervous. The more he tried to put it out of his mind, the more it nagged at him.

By 9:00 P.M., Alisha had already been making none-too-subtle suggestions about going to bed early for a half hour or more. She grew even more insistent after her parents said good night and headed upstairs a short time later, but Larry kept stalling and making excuses until after the ten o'clock news on TV.

"There's a late movie on Channel 7 that sounds pretty good," he said. "I thought I might check it out."

Alisha frowned at him, her eyes flashing warning signals. "I get the feeling you're trying to avoid me, Larry," she said.

"Don't be silly," he protested. "I'm just not sleepy, that's all."

She moved close to him and pressed her lips to his ear. "I'm not *sleepy,* either, lover," she breathed. "But I *am* ready to go to bed, if you catch my drift."

As Larry switched off the TV and followed her, a powerful surge of desire raced through him. Halfway up the stairs, he caught up with her and threw his arms around her. A minute later, they were in the bedroom with the door closed behind them, and he could feel his erection swelling.

Then he distinctly heard Alisha's mother's voice, telling Alisha's father to put down his book and turn out the lamp. Her words were as audible as if she were right there in the same room with them instead of on the other side of the wall. Alisha's father mumbled something in reply, and Larry heard the sound of the book being closed and plopped down on a bedside table, then the click of the lamp.

Larry felt an abrupt sense of panic. These walls must be as thin as paper, he thought.

In the time it took for the thought to form, Larry's erection had vanished. Long after Alisha had turned petulantly away from him and gone to sleep, he lay there staring at the ceiling and wondering what had happened.

Exposing Hidden Conflicts

The kind of performance anxiety that sprang from Larry's fear of being overheard by Alisha's parents as he made love to Alisha is relatively common and readily understandable. A lot of men would feel tense and unable to relax in this sort of situation. A sizable percentage of them might be strongly enough affected to experience temporary erectile problems.

I explained this to Larry when he finally came to me more than a year later. By then, though, the scenario had repeated itself ten or twelve times. The outcome was always identical and had become grimly predictable. Never once was Larry able to maintain an erection sufficient for intercourse while he was in that bedroom at his in-laws' house, yet he had no difficulty whatsoever when he was back in his own home again.

The problem was compounded by Alisha's determined insistence that he keep trying each time they visited her parents. This was harder to understand than Larry's problem.

"It was really bad at Thanksgiving and Christmas, when we spent a total of seven nights there," Larry lamented. "I kept telling Alisha it wouldn't work, but she wouldn't listen. She kept trying different things, but nothing really helped. I said, 'Look, can't we just lay off for a few days and then make up for lost time when we get back to our own place?' And she said, 'No, damn it, I want to do it *here.*' It sounds crazy, but I swear to God I think she's going to divorce me if I don't figure out how to have sex with her at her parents' house."

This remark provided some fresh insight into how Alisha might be contributing to the problem, and I asked Larry to bring her with him to our next session. After talking with both of them, I managed to uncover the hidden conflict that was creating barriers between them and threatening their relationship.

As a seventh grader, Larry had once been caught in an embarrassing situation with a slightly younger girl who lived next door. The girl's parents had returned home unexpectedly and found the two of them together in her bedroom, not actually having sex yet but very close to that point. Larry described it as the most frightening, disturbing incident of his life. The girl's father had told Larry's parents, and Larry had been humiliated, reprimanded, and denied privileges for months afterward as punishment.

Within the security of his own domicile, Larry could function very well sexually, but the boyhood incident had left him with a deep-seated fear of something like that happening again in someone else's house. Consequently, each time he heard Alisha's parents moving or talking in the next room—or even thought about them being there so close by—it triggered his embarrassment and anxiety all over again.

Alisha, meanwhile, was besieged by an opposing set of emotional forces. She harbored a burning resentment against her narrow-minded, superstrict parents, who had refused to let her go on a single date all through high school. She had never even been allowed to sit with a boy in church or visit with one on the front porch in the middle of the afternoon.

Now that she was married and beyond their control, she had a perverse subconscious urge to flaunt her sexuality in the faces of her parents, to rub their noses in it, so to speak. She enjoyed defying their cold morality by openly kissing and rubbing herself against Larry in their presence, but that wasn't enough. Alisha didn't care in the least if her parents heard ecstatic moans or bedsprings creaking from the room next to theirs. On the contrary, she *wanted* them to.

The very thought of her mother and father listening helplessly to the explicit sounds of her having an orgasm with Larry aroused Alisha tremendously, and she was infuriated when he was unable to help her satisfy this compulsive, long-suppressed urge.

Finding the Best Medicine

Even if it had been available at the time, I have grave doubts that Viagra would have improved Larry and Alisha's basic relationship. True, it would have enabled them to hook up the plumbing and allowed Alisha to act out her bitterness against her parents. But the relationship would still have been flawed and limited by immature emotions, self-centeredness, and a lack of spontaneity. The hidden conflicts would remain unresolved, and they would most likely resurface to do more harm in the future.

As it turned out, that's precisely what happened.

In a psychiatric sense, reassurance is the best "medicine" for performance anxiety, and when I explained to Larry that many men would have similar problems in similar circumstances, he regained a measure of his lost self-confidence. Understanding how his current difficulties related to his traumatic long-ago experience as a boy also helped to some extent. But if they hoped to take their relationship to a more mature level, I knew that both Alisha and Larry had a lot of sexual and emotional growing up to do.

I strongly recommended additional psychotherapy, but once Larry overcame his dysfunction well enough to fulfill Alisha's fantasy of having sex in her parents' house, they discontinued their sessions. Within two years, each of them became involved in an extramarital affair, and their marriage ended in divorce.

What role could Viagra have played in altering this scenario for the better? Not a very meaningful one, I'm afraid. There's little doubt that Larry's immediate difficulty could have been resolved more rapidly with the drug, but I seriously doubt that it would have changed the situation's eventual unhappy outcome. Viagra simply wouldn't have been the best medicine in this case. But what else is there to be learned here?

For one thing, some people are more bothered by situational factors than others. Although Larry couldn't feel comfortable enough to have sex in a bedroom that adjoined his in-laws', other men could perform in the display window of Saks Fifth Avenue at five o'clock in the afternoon. What is a critical situational factor for one person may amount to nothing for another. Alisha, for example, wasn't bothered at all. In fact, the situation played right into her neurotic need to flaunt her sexuality in front of, or at least in earshot of, her parents.

To be successful, the treatment focus would have had to be different for Larry and Alisha. For Larry, the right therapy would have been reassurance, not pills; it would be important for Larry to respect his own feelings about a place he found inappropriate for sex. For Alisha, the treatment goal (if she had decided to be a patient) would have been for her to confront her destructive behavior and try to understand what earlier unresolved needs were fueling it.

A Healthy Dose of Guilt

Although Larry was with his own wife, his experiences at his in-laws' house weren't much different, in a sense, from those encountered every day by countless errant husbands. It's a familiar story, one that often goes something like this:

A married businessman attends an out-of-town convention, leaving his wife and kids at home and spending four or five nights alone in a strange city. Under ordinary circumstances, this man is an upstanding citizen, a devoted husband, and a loving father who would never do anything to betray his family's trust.

But as the convention wears on, loneliness sets in, and the obligatory daily phone call home does nothing to dispel it. The man meets an attractive woman who is also alone, and one thing leads predictably to another. They go to dinner together, then linger to talk, and both drink a bit too much. He walks her back to her hotel, and she invites him up to her room. Almost before he realizes it, they're in bed together.

And then . . . nothing happens.

At the critical moment, visions of his wife and children flash hauntingly in the man's mind, followed in rapid succession by (1) chilling guilt, (2) numbing anxiety, and (3) sudden erectile failure. A psychological bucket of ice water douses the fire in his loins and leaves him as limp as a boiled noodle.

"Dear God," he thinks, "what am I *doing?*"

He mutters an inept apology to the woman, jumps out of bed, frantically pulls his clothes on—and flees.

As far as the man's sexual dysfunction is concerned, this is merely another case of being in the wrong place at the wrong time. The diagnosis is the same—performance anxiety—and so is the result.

But in this instance, a healthy dose of guilt has spared this man a painful load of remorse and self-blame that he might otherwise carry for the rest of his life.

Now let's suppose for a moment that this same man swallows a potency pill when he first begins to sense the direction in which the evening is heading. Beyond question, he feels the same sense of guilt, yet now, instead of being physically unable to perform, he has a fully functional erection. Unless he also has exceptional willpower, the man may very well end up going through with the sex act in spite of his misgivings.

Would you want Viagra at your disposal in a similar situation? Before you answer that question, remember that a number of men suffer fatal heart attacks each year during exactly this sort of illicit liaison, so a definite element of risk exists in using a potency drug in such circumstances. One study showed a sharp increase in risk among middle-aged men who indulged in a heavy meal and alcohol and who were with an unfamiliar partner in an unfamiliar setting.

So, should a physician simply give this conventioner a pill and a pat on the back and tell him to try again? Not in my book. This man's penis has more sense than he has. His impulse to cheat may be a sign of dissatisfaction in his marriage, but it's always better to talk to a health care professional about these kinds of feelings than to act them out with strangers.

If I gave this man Viagra or any other similar pill that comes along, I would be doing nothing to help him resolve his real underlying problem—and I might be exposing him to an increased risk of death.

Living and Learning

While the mating urge is instinctive in all creatures, sex between human beings is largely learned behavior. No one is born knowing how to make love, much less how to deal with all the emotional stimuli that relate to sexual relationships. It takes years of physical maturization before a person is capable of functioning sexually, and it frequently takes far longer to attain the level of psychological maturity that can sustain a relationship for a lifetime.

One of the major theories around which modern sex therapy revolves is one popularized by Masters and Johnson in the 1970s, although behavior therapists were aware of it much earlier than that. The theory holds that sexual dysfunction occurs when some negative aspect is paired with the sexual experience and/or when arousal is counteracted by anxiety.

We can see these two forces at work in the experiences of both Larry H. and the lonely conventioneer. In addition, these dysfunctions were aggravated by the fact that one relationship was, for all practical purposes, meaningless, and the other was marred by immaturity on the part of both partners.

In their study *Human Sexual Inadequacy,* published in 1970, Masters and Johnson concluded that the relationship itself can be the source of the dysfunction. Some unresolved issue between the partners can subvert and undermine their sexual response and performance. This isn't in the nature of a deep-rooted unconscious conflict but in a simple misalignment, such as the one that affected Martin and Betty L.

When the couple has a strong, mature relationship, as Martin and Betty did, simple relaxation exercises or small changes in routine can often help them work through the dysfunction.

In less mature relationships, such as Larry and Alisha's, it may also be possible to remove the symptoms but extremely difficult to achieve anything that could be classified as a cure.

In my view, curing dysfunction amounts to more than just neutralizing a patient's anxiety enough for him to perform sexually, whether it's done with a pill or psychotherapy. A true cure comes only when both parties are able to make accommodations to keep improving their relationship and finding mature ways to relate to each other.

How sexually mature are you? When you have intercourse, what's most important to you about the experience? If your own gratification always comes first, give yourself a low score on the maturity scale. But if your partner's pleasure and the feelings of togetherness and shared intimacy are major priorities for you, it means you're "growing up" sexually.

When that happens, certain times and places may still be better than others, but the total sexual experience can become an overwhelmingly positive one.

8
Learned and Social Factors

The gender-equality movement of the past quarter century has gone a long way toward blurring the traditional boundary lines between the sexes, changing even the traditional concepts of what is "masculine" and "feminine" in character. But the psychological barriers between the sexes are considerably more difficult to eliminate than the economic, political, and institutional ones. There are compelling reasons to doubt whether men and women will ever achieve sameness in the way they think, feel, and react to life's essential situations and relationships—or, for that matter, whether they *should* achieve it.

When it comes to sexuality and the basic human functions that spring from it—reproduction, parenting, nest building, and the process that we call loving—men and women are still very different, and they probably always will be. The so-called war between the sexes, which dates back tens of thousands of years, has definitely entered a new phase in recent times, one in which the male is no longer automatically dominant. Yet the elemental emotional conflicts that started the war are still there. They may be more complex or subtle in their modern context, but they may also be more intense.

Today's typical young father changes far more diapers than did his predecessors of thirty or forty years ago, and a typical young mother is much more likely to leave her baby in day care to compete with men in the job market. But in their sexual roles, they still carry much of the same emotional baggage as their great-great-grandparents. They are instinctively programmed that way, and no amount of legislated equality is likely to change that programming. It will probably require generations of experiencing and re-experiencing new roles and learning and accepting new behavior patterns for such fundamental change to take place.

In the meantime, the ongoing struggle for sexual identity creates a fertile climate for sexual dysfunction.

A Pair of Albatrosses

Stamped into the psychological makeup of modern man and modern woman are age-old sexual identities that clash violently with much of what our present society teaches each to expect. In many ways, these identities are like a pair of emotional albatrosses hanging around their respective necks. In its own way, each albatross contributes materially to the impotency epidemic in this country.

Modern man, who now shares a considerable measure of his former power with women, is nonetheless still pressed by his emotions to be autonomous, strong, and independent. They instill in him the ideal of pulling himself up by his own bootstraps, even if he's never worn boots in his life.

It is generally much harder, for example, for a man to go to a doctor than it is for a woman. In their movies, Harrison Ford and Arnold Schwarzenegger sew up their own wounds, and although Clint Eastwood cried in one of his recent films, I doubt that you'll ever see him or Bruce Willis portrayed as a person seeking help for a sexual problem.

Men of the 1990s *are* more sensitive than their counterparts of past generations, but the albatross still urges modern man to walk tall and proud. Young guys still wear T-shirts that say "No Fear" and train themselves not to show visible signs of weakness.

So when sexual dysfunction strikes, modern man often refuses to accept the fact that he can't solve his problem on his own. To do otherwise would be to admit to being vulnerable, maybe even frightened and confused, and this would be an obvious sign of weakness. Consequently, when his wife suggests that he see a doctor about the sexual difficulties that are making his life an agony, modern man still often covers up his true feelings with hostility and rage.

Like his ancestors, he may flare: "I don't need a damned doctor. I can work it out by myself."

In other words, even with a limp penis, he feels the need to maintain a stiff upper lip.

Some modern women, meanwhile, also carry their own leftover albatross from another time. They are much more outwardly independent, but they often feel the same deep-seated need for love and approval that ruled the emotions and actions of their ancient counterparts. Today's woman is generally more forthright than her mother would have been in trying to get her man to confront his problem, but in many cases she doesn't want to be too pushy or critical, for fear of alienating him. This often inhibits her in dealing with sexual issues with her partner. This may sound outdated, but I continue to see this as a factor for many of the women who consult me about sexual problems.

Ingrained emotions and behavioral patterns die hard. This same fear still keeps these women from letting their men know what they want and don't want sexually or from complaining about being sexually shortchanged. Women are typically much more patient than men with conditions that are imperfect, uncomfortable, distressing, or even downright miserable.

Patience can be a genuine virtue, but it can be carried to extremes when a woman is afraid of "rocking the boat." Showing too much patience and forbearance has been known to cost women their lives at the hands of abusive males, when they refused to leave or call the police after repeated beatings. It can also allow severe sexual problems to drag on for far too long.

Women Take the Initiative

Fortunately, a growing number of today's women are able to throw off their albatross and take the initiative in dealing with male sexual problems.

Since the advent of Viagra, a huge percentage of those who have besieged physicians' offices with calls for information about the drug have been the wives and lovers of men who were too stubborn or embarrassed to make the call themselves. In my opinion, these women deserve a lot of credit for taking a crucial step toward strengthening their relationships and improving their own sexual experiences along with those of their mates.

That's why, when a woman contacts me about her husband's sexual difficulties—as many have over the years—and begs me not to let him know what she's doing, I always respect her confidence. In numerous instances, I've consulted initially with the wife alone, then helped her determine the best way to broach the subject with her husband.

"Hardheaded Henry"

I've treated and counseled many couples who had fallen victim to those emotional albatrosses of social or learned behavior, but one particular case in which treatment was initiated by the woman always springs to mind. It involved a man whom I still think of as "hardheaded Henry" and his long-suffering wife, Eileen.

When Eileen first called me, Henry had already been having sexual difficulties for at least ten years, but they had recently become more severe. At first, her story sounded much like dozens of others I had dealt with in the past, but it soon became evident that certain factors placed this situation in a special category.

What Eileen told me on her initial visit to my office had a decidedly familiar ring to it. She was thirty-four and her husband was thirty-six. He was an assistant football coach at a large parochial high school, an avid exercise enthusiast who ran and lifted weights four or five times a week, and a man who took great pride in his physical conditioning and bulging muscles. He also fit the feminists' definition of a "chauvinist pig" if anyone ever did.

"Henry would probably never forgive me if he knew I was here—much less if he heard what I was saying," she began nervously. "But in all the time we've been together, he's hardly ever satisfied me sexually. There's just no other way to put it, and to make things even worse, he doesn't seem to care if I get anything out of our lovemaking or not."

"Are you saying that you don't have orgasms?" I asked.

She shook her head vehemently. "Not in years. I've had three children with Henry, but I could literally count the number of orgasms I've had since we got married on the fingers of one hand. I keep thinking there's got to be something we can do to make things better, but if anything, it just keeps getting worse. I'd never be unfaithful to Henry, but sometimes I can't help thinking . . ."

"What goes wrong when you and your husband have intercourse?" I asked. "Can you describe what happens?"

Talking about the intimate details of her sexual experiences with Henry made Eileen very uncomfortable, and it took her quite a while to provide complete answers to my questions. Finally, though, she made it clear that Henry had no difficulty getting an erection, but it never lasted long enough for his wife to reach orgasm. He was ejaculating much too quickly and losing his erection within a few seconds after penetration.

Henry wasn't suffering from erectile dysfunction but from premature ejaculation, another very common type of male sexual problem, which patients sometimes mistake for impotence and which can, in some cases, lead to erectile dysfunction.

"I know it'll be hard to do," I told Eileen, "but I hope you'll go home and tell your husband exactly what you've told me. Then, if you can get him to agree, I'd like to see the two of you together."

"I'll do the best I can," she said, but she didn't sound optimistic.

Surprisingly, though, she phoned three days later to make an appointment for her husband and herself. I didn't find out until much later that Henry had agreed to come in only after she threatened to take the children and leave unless he did. Eileen was tougher than she looked or acted, and it was good that she was. She was going to need all the fortitude she could muster in dealing with "hard-headed Henry" over the next month or so.

For the most part, Henry was sullen and silent during our initial session. His pride was obviously injured, and I think he was genuinely stunned by his wife's complaints and assertiveness, which I'm sure seemed totally out of character after all the years she had spent acquiescing to him. But at least he gave the appearance of listening to what was being said, and he didn't get up and storm out.

Who's in Charge Here?

As the therapy continued, I was able to trace the origins of Henry's premature ejaculations back to his teenage years. Like many other adolescents of his generation, Henry's first experiences with sexual intercourse had been of what I call the "bang-bang" variety: The scene was often the backseat of a car at the drive-in movies. The girl was invariably nervous and afraid of being spotted by a security patrolman or someone she knew. The boy was bumbling and awkward but determined to finish what he had started. Masters and Johnson believe that many young men who start out with this sort of initiation to sexual intercourse have a tendency to rush matters in later life as well.

Like his parents before him, Henry was also a devout Catholic who took all the sex-related tenets of his religion very much to heart. He was adamantly opposed to all types of artificial birth-control devices, but he saw nothing wrong with withdrawing his penis a split second before ejaculation in an effort to prevent sperm from entering his partner's vagina. This, too, added to his hurry-hurry attitude toward intercourse and made him still more prone to ejaculate prematurely.

One of the most common therapies for premature ejaculation is known as the "stop and start" technique, in which the couple initiates intercourse but then pauses before the man can reach orgasm and lose his erection. In this technique, the man lies on his back with the woman astride him, and she basically controls the situation.

In their first session with me after I recommended this therapy, I could tell that things weren't going well between Henry and Eileen. She seemed agitated, and she kept "looking daggers" at her husband, while he was more huffy and noncommittal than ever. That was the day, by the way, that Eileen bestowed his well-deserved nickname on Henry.

"You're just being hardheaded," she told him as they walked into my office. "You're just not cooperating at all."

"What's the trouble?" I asked.

"I don't like that new technique," Henry muttered after a long pause. "It's not right for the woman to be on top and the guy to be on the bottom. It makes me feel like some kind of freak. I mean, it's not natural—not the way God intended."

While admitting that I claimed no ability to read God's mind, I tried to explain that, at least to my knowledge, no religious rule or statutory law prohibits a man from lying on his back with his partner above him during intercourse.

"If it helps you keep an erection longer and makes intercourse more satisfying," I said, "what difference does it make?"

"It's just not . . . not *manly*," he finally sputtered.

Actually, of course, Henry's real reason for opposing the therapy was his reluctance to let his wife control the tempo of their lovemaking. To him, the man was always supposed to take the lead and be in charge, and the woman was supposed to follow along, whether she liked it or not. It was more of the same selfish attitude that had been contributing to the problem between this couple all along.

When I suggested an exercise in which the woman massages the man's genitals until he is fully aroused, but the couple stops short of actual intercourse, Henry again objected, this time citing strong religious reservations. Church doctrine, he argued, holds that any sexual act performed willingly by a married couple is acceptable—but only as long as it ends in intercourse. In his view, this exercise failed to meet that criterion.

"I can't do it," he said flatly. "It's against my religion."

A Decisive Turnaround

At this point, I was beginning to get a bit frustrated myself with "hardheaded Henry," but not nearly as frustrated as Eileen. As I was trying to explain that the exercise would, indeed, lead to intercourse eventually, although possibly not in the same day, she leaned forward and slammed her fist down on the arm of the couch.

She made no effort to hide the fury in her voice. "Divorce is against your religion, too, Henry, so you'd better quit finding fault with everything the doctor suggests and start being sensible. If you don't, I swear the next appointment I make is going to be with a lawyer. I mean it, Henry."

Henry looked as if his wife had just slapped him in the face—and she looked as if she wanted to do exactly that.

I spent the rest of the session trying to defuse the anger between them and offer some calming reassurance. But as the couple left that day, I couldn't help feeling pessimistic about their chances of resolving their problem. Some flexibility on Henry's part was absolutely essential, and I wasn't sure he was capable of it. Now his stubborn resistance was bringing counter-resistance from Eileen. They seemed further apart than ever, and it didn't look hopeful.

Surprisingly, though, that day marked the beginning of a decisive turnaround for Henry and Eileen. For all his hardheadedness, Henry honestly valued his marriage and family, and he had been deeply shaken by his wife's angry outburst—shaken enough to listen to reason for once. His reluctance to try the recommended exercises and therapies eased after Eileen convinced him there was nothing "sinful" about them and persuaded him to relax and devote more time to their lovemaking.

Just a couple of weeks later, Eileen reported her first orgasm in at least three years. After that, orgasms became increasingly routine for her, and she and Henry found pleasure and fulfillment in sexual intimacy that they had never experienced before.

As the therapy added to their arousal and desire, they also made another discovery: Even if Henry ejaculated prematurely the first time they had intercourse, he could get a second erection within about thirty minutes with stimulation from his wife. Since it normally takes a man longer to reach orgasm a second successive time than it did the first time, the problem was much less likely to recur when they had intercourse again within a short period.

In finally being able to give his wife true sexual satisfaction, Henry felt reassured about his "manliness," and it no longer mattered who was on the top or the bottom. But more important, he also discovered a level of satisfaction he had never known before. When Henry "grew up" sexually, he also enabled the relationship to grow richer and more mature.

There are medications specifically designed to delay orgasm, but I seriously doubt that giving Henry such a drug would have played a constructive role in overcoming the problem between him and Eileen. Prescribing Viagra was another consideration. Although it hasn't been shown to relieve premature ejaculation, Viagra might have shortened Henry's refractory period, so that he could more easily and quickly have intercourse a second time.

But I felt that using Viagra in this case could also have had distinct liabilities that might have weakened this marriage, rather than strengthening it. Once Eileen made her sexual dissatisfaction known, the relationship entered a crucial stage. At this point, Henry's ego and machismo could easily have motivated him to seek out other partners who might have been less critical of his performance, at least openly. Viagra or any other simple solution might merely have facilitated that destructive search.

I decided that joint counseling was the most effective way to improve this couple's troubled sex life. As it turned out, the right answer turned out to be extensive "couple work," not just popping a pill.

Are your concepts of what constitutes "proper" sexual practices too narrow and rigid for your own good? My advice to couples is to be willing to keep searching and experimenting until they find what's right for them. Flexibility and mutual caring are frequently the primary keys to better sexual experiences and more rewarding relationships.

I don't think anyone should have to do anything sexually that he or she finds upsetting. But on the other hand, I also believe that condemning something you've never tried can be a costly mistake.

How do you know if you've been unduly influenced by learned or social factors that can inhibit sexual performance or interfere with solving a sexual problem? If your responses are stereotypical, preprogrammed, or "automatic," consider that a danger signal. An example is Henry's idea that real men don't have intercourse while lying on their backs. Says who? This idea usually grows out of confusion over concepts of active roles versus passive ones. In the mind of the affected man, it works something like this: Women are passive. Therefore their sexual role is to be on their backs.

Actually, one's position during intercourse has very little to do with being passive or active. Healthy, well-adjusted partners can take turns in playing the passive and active roles without posing a threat to either.

Another example: Men should initiate sex. Says who? That makes no more sense than a woman always waiting to eat until her partner tells her he's hungry. Either partner can initiate sex, and either partner has the right to veto it. These powers don't reside in one gender or the other.

Another example: A man should know what a woman likes sexually, and the woman should never have to tell him. Since when? Men are not experts in what excites women. Each woman is an expert in what excites her individually. The same goes for men. Men and women need to learn what satisfies their partners by asking them about their needs.

Another example: My religion forbids me to (fill in the blank). This is among the toughest forms of learned or social behavior to overcome. I usually ask the person to cite chapter and verse and consult with their priest, minister, or rabbi about specifics. It generally turns out that the person's religious interpretations are highly individualized, without much basis in actual religious doctrine, and are often used as rationalizations to avoid issues that frighten them. Masters and Johnson found that the deeper the religious prohibition is ingrained in the patient's mind, however, the higher the odds against getting him or her to change.

Learned Taboos Versus Reality

"Hardheaded Henry" was by no means the only individual whose learned restrictions and cultural taboos clashed with the reality of his sexual needs. A Jewish rabbi once consulted me about erectile dysfunction. He had very little direct knowledge of his own sexual responses, since touching his penis wasn't permitted under his religious views. Therefore, he was unable to tell me if he had erections when he masturbated because he wasn't able to masturbate.

Millions of people in every walk of life are conditioned by social influences and learned behavior to assume unrealistic sexual attitudes and practices. Sometimes, the conditioning is subtle and gradual, sometimes sudden and violent.

Countless women suffer from hypoactive (abnormally low) sexual desire. Some are rape victims for whom sex has become an ugly, dehumanizing experience. Some are married to wife beaters for whom they have lost all feelings except fear and loathing. Others have been brainwashed through an unreasonably strict upbringing to reject sex as "dirty" and distasteful.

Following the birth of a child, a wife may come to view her husband as a father image, or a husband may start identifying his wife as his mother. In either case, this can lead to sexual alienation because we've all been taught that father-daughter, mother-son sex is immoral and abhorrent. In counseling couples, I've come across any number of cases where both the husband and the wife had been conditioned to fear or avoid sexual contact by learned or social influences that neither one was able to recognize, much less cope with.

Paul and Della R. were just such a couple. They had been married for more than twenty-five years, but for close to half that period their sexual relationship had been virtually nonexistent. For a while, the more I learned about the barriers between them, the more I doubted that they could ever be warm and loving toward each other. I was very gratified when they proved me wrong.

An Emotional Wasteland

Paul was fifty-three, the president of a small trucking company. He seemed quiet and mild-mannered when he and Della first came to my office, but surface impressions can be deceiving. Experience had taught me long ago never to "judge a book by its cover," yet I was surprised to learn, during the course of joint and individual therapy sessions with the couple, that Paul was actually a very abusive person. Not only was he prone to fits of temper but, according to Della, he had also slapped her and pushed her around dozens of times over the years, particularly when he was younger.

For a decade or more, Paul had been bothered by mild to moderate erectile dysfunction, and his sexual difficulties had intensified the abuse he heaped on Della. He was angry and resentful, and he made it clear that he blamed her for the problem, although he never explained why. When she tried to offer encouragement or sympathy, it only made matters worse. He continued to attempt to have intercourse with her at regular intervals of about once a month, and when he was unable to perform—as was often the case—he would fly into a rage. Sometimes he would curse her and bodily push her off the bed onto the floor. Other times, he would charge through the house, breaking things and overturning furniture, then barricade himself in the guest bedroom for the rest of the night. Occasionally, he would drive off in the car and not come back until the next day.

"Those were very lonely, hellish years for me," Della confided. "I thought a thousand times about leaving, but I had no place to go, so I just let it drag on and on. I kept hoping that someday, somehow Paul would change and we could go back to being the way we were when we first got together. He was more considerate then, and he tried harder to keep a rein on his temper."

Finding Courage in Crisis

It took a grim turn of events to trigger the change in Paul for which Della had hoped for so long. When she was forty-nine, Della was diagnosed with uterine cancer and had to have a total hysterectomy. The ordeal frightened and depressed her, but it also gave her a strong new resolve to do something about the emotional wasteland that her marriage had become.

"All of a sudden, I found courage I never knew I had before," she said. "For the first time in my life, I was able to stand up to Paul and tell him I wasn't going to live like this anymore."

Most amazingly of all, considering how little outward concern he had shown for Della for such a long time, his wife's illness left Paul even more anxious and unnerved than she was. When he visited her in the hospital after the surgery, he sat on the edge of her bed and tears actually ran down his cheeks. Della had never seen him cry before.

"Don't you go and die on me now," he whispered. "I couldn't stand it if you did."

"Unless our life together gets better," she told him bluntly, "I don't feel like I have much reason to live."

Later, when she came home, the marked change in Paul's demeanor toward Della continued. He almost seemed to be a different person. Now he was always quiet and solicitous, no longer blustering or raising his voice to her—much less his hand. He waited on her attentively and uncomplainingly, fixing her meals and doing household chores that he had never volunteered to do before. He even put aside his business responsibilities to spend extra time at home with her.

For several months during her recuperation, Della completely lost her desire for sex. Even after she recovered physically from the surgery, she went through a period of deep depression, a fairly common symptom among women following a hysterectomy, which made it virtually impossible for her to become aroused. Once her estrogen levels were properly regulated and her doctor prescribed an antidepressant for her, however, Della began to feel better. She was also buoyed by the change in her husband, and her interest in sex started to return.

Now, though, there was another problem. Whenever she tried to initiate sexual contact with Paul, he shied away. He was unfailingly considerate otherwise, but it soon became apparent that he was avoiding her sexually, and Della couldn't figure out why. Even during the years when he was cursing her and blaming her for his erectile difficulties, he had never acted like this.

When she asked him what was wrong, she could sense him withdrawing still further and retreating into a kind of shell. To try to reassure him, she told him not to worry about getting an erection, that feeling warmth and closeness between them was the important thing to her, but it didn't seem to do any good. Once, when she pressed him on the subject, he even burst into tears.

The relationship was still at this peculiar stalemate when Della finally convinced Paul to join her in psychotherapy. When I was able to talk to him individually and delve into his early background, the source of both his past and present sexual problems was finally revealed.

A Lingering Tragedy

When Paul was ten years old, his mother died of cancer. He was never told any of the medical details of her illness, but he recalled veiled references being made to its effecting her "female parts," and he was pretty sure it was either uterine or cervical cancer. At any rate, his mother's death was the worst tragedy of Paul's life, and he had never recovered from the sense of emptiness and loss it left him with. He still had vivid memories of being taken into his mother's hospital room to say good-bye and of his father sitting at her bedside sobbing uncontrollably. It was the first time he'd ever seen a grown man weep.

This traumatic loss had shattered his world and left Paul, the boy, with deep-seated feelings of weakness and insecurity—feelings that Paul, the man, would later try to cover up with outward displays of hostility and abusiveness.

When, like his mother, Della was stricken with cancer, Paul, the man, could no longer suppress the terror and anxiety of Paul, the boy, and it all came churning to the surface. It was like reliving the horror of that childhood experience all over again, and it made Paul determined to do everything in his power to keep from losing Della the way he had lost his mother.

But in this process, Della became, in effect, a substitute mother, rather than a wife. When Paul made this psychological transition, the idea of having sex with Della became repellent to him. In his mind, it would have been the same as committing incest with his mother. (I'll discuss this phenomenon in greater detail in an upcoming chapter on the intrapsychic factors that often impact sexual function.)

For a time, Paul had become totally impotent, but there was no physical basis for his impotency. From the earliest signs of mild erectile dysfunction, his problem had always been psychogenic in nature. To put it as simply as possible, if he thought about losing his mother during sexual arousal or intercourse, it had an immediate negative effect on his performance. If he distracted himself sufficiently by showing anger and hostility toward his wife, his performance improved, but a pattern of abuse also developed.

With continued psychotherapy, Paul and Della were able to forge a stronger, more mutually satisfying relationship than they had ever known before—or ever dreamed of knowing, for that matter. It wasn't idyllic by any means, but few long-term relationships are. The point is that she became more assertive, and he became less hostile. At long last, the abuse and fear that had marred their relationship for many years ended, and they were finally able to enjoy sex in a blame-free, nonconfrontational atmosphere.

As I said earlier, considering the depth and duration of their difficulties, I was pleasantly surprised.

Would a "potency pill" have allowed Paul to get an erection? Early on, the answer would almost certainly have been "yes." But later, when his impotency and sexual avoidance became more severe, I'm not so sure. Even with Viagra, if the man can't be stimulated sufficiently, nothing will happen, and Paul faced a formidable mental barrier to arousal.

But the larger question is whether or not an oral drug would have enabled this couple to confront and overcome the complex psychological problems that threatened their relationship. The answer to that is certainly *not*.

What can you learn from this case? Traumatic events in themselves have little meaning. Each person experiences the trauma differently. For Della, her surgery was a red badge of courage that enabled her to stand up to Paul for the first time in their marriage. For Paul, his wife's hysterectomy rekindled old unresolved issues about his mother's death that caused him to regress emotionally.

In such cases, the sexual symptom is like the tip of an iceberg. It's the ticket that gets the patient into my office in the first place, and this is good. But as I'm reminded every day in my practice, it isn't just the sex that's important. It's also the relationship.

9 Larger Psychiatric Problems

Sexual dysfunction is often merely a physical manifestation of a much larger, more pervasive psychiatric problem, such as clinical depression, bipolar disorder (manic depression), or psychosis. When it is, treating the larger problem should always be given priority over the sexual dysfunction. A drug like Viagra might well relieve the dysfunction itself, but giving it to such a patient without first dealing with the larger psychiatric problem can be compared to treating a compound fracture with a Band-Aid or trying to put out a forest fire with a water pistol.

Giving Viagra to a man with severe undiagnosed depression could be a huge and potentially disastrous medical mistake. A patient suffering from severe depression frequently poses a danger to himself. Suicidal tendencies are one of the hallmark symptoms of depression, and in some circumstances a suicidal man with an erection could be more unstable than a suicidal man without one.

The possibility of danger in this kind of situation worries me. It's another vitally important reason why physicians should not take the quick-and-easy approach to Viagra and why they should evaluate every patient carefully before the drug is prescribed.

In depression, libido is usually among the first things to go and one of the last to come back. Without libido, there can be no interest in sexual stimulation, and without stimulation, there can be no erection. Therefore, when a man is severely depressed, it's questionable how much benefit he can gain from Viagra anyway. But even if an erection should result, treating a sex problem without addressing an underlying cause still accomplishes nothing.

Missing the Big Picture

I've treated hundreds of cases of depression during my career, but none was more fascinating or dramatic than the one involving Douglas F., a fifty-year-old insurance executive. By most people's standards, Doug was quite wealthy and successful. He was also handsome, distinguished, charming, articulate, and debonair, and I'm sure he was admired and even envied by many of his friends and business associates.

They might have felt differently toward him, however, if they had known how inwardly troubled and tormented he was. Doug very nearly had the dubious distinction of going through two marriages without once having vaginal intercourse with either of his wives. In my view, that would be enough to depress any man—and Doug *was* severely depressed.

When he finally found his way to me, Doug had been wandering for months among a half dozen different physicians, each of whom was attempting to treat him for some isolated ailment. He consulted one doctor for persistent digestive upsets, another for chronic exhaustion, another for insomnia, another for headaches, and so on.

One of the most perplexing problems in today's highly technical and largely depersonalized health care system springs from the fact that the overwhelming majority of physicians are now specialists. Their expertise is often confined to one narrow area of medicine or even one small part of the body. Psychiatry, of course, is one of the world's oldest medical specialties, so I certainly can't fault other physicians for entering special fields of their own. But unlike some specialists in other fields, I recognize the fact that the problems I treat can affect many parts of the body, and in my practice I make every effort to view and treat each individual patient as a whole person.

My point is that, too often, specialists may not be able to "see the forest for the trees." They are intensely familiar with one disease process or one family of diseases and highly knowledgeable in the latest methods of treating them. Yet they may not be nearly as adept at grasping the "big picture" of the entire human organism as are many of the general practitioners who rank well below the specialists in medicine's professional pecking order. An ear, nose, and throat specialist, for example, may know all there is to know about sinuses but have only a general working knowledge of the urinary system.

This piecemeal approach compounded the situation in which Doug found himself. Since he could afford the very best treatment, he naturally sought out specialists for each of his complaints. Each time a new complaint developed, he consulted a different specialist. Each doctor prescribed a drug that he believed would be beneficial, then sent Doug on his way.

Meanwhile, all of Doug's physical upsets and nagging pains were real enough to him, yet every last one of them was a by-product of his depression. It was only after he remarked offhandedly to one of his doctors that he sometimes thought about suicide that the physician referred Doug to me.

A Marriage Without Sex

The first time I talked to him, Doug was calm and rational enough, but he also seemed listless, subdued, and almost unconcerned about his condition. This isn't unusual for a severely depressed person, especially one who has lived with depression constantly for years. Many such people reach the point where they expect to feel bad and have something wrong with them all the time. They give up on ever feeling comfortable or content, much less happy. This resignation becomes hopelessness, which often leads to thoughts of suicide.

Diagnosing Doug's depression was the easy part. Treating it effectively was an entirely different story. I prescribed Prozac for him and advised him to discontinue all the other prescription medications he was taking, at least for the time being. Within a few weeks, this powerful antidepressant could be expected to elevate Doug's mood and help him function better—and I suspected it would also relieve many of his physical complaints. But if he was actually going to overcome the depression, rather than just holding it in check, it was important to track down its origins and try to eliminate the cause.

One of the first questions I asked Doug during our initial session was, "Are you married?"

"Yes," he said, "my first wife died four years ago, and I remarried last September." (That would have been approximately ten months earlier.)

"And how's the new marriage working out?"

He shrugged. "Oh, all right, I guess," he said vaguely.

"How often do you and your present wife have sexual intercourse?" I asked.

"We don't," he said without a trace of emotion. "We never have."

"You've been married all this time, and you've never had intercourse? Why?"

"I guess because neither one of us is that interested in it. We tried a few times, but I wasn't able to do anything, so we just gave up on it. I figure, what the hell, why fight it? What difference does it make?"

"What does your wife think about this?" I asked. "Doesn't it make a difference to her?"

Doug shrugged again. "I don't know," he said. "I never asked her."

A Bizarre Story Unfolds

Doug's admission of impotency came as no great surprise, considering the severity of his depression, and I was reasonably sure that it was directly related to a loss of libido, but until that conversation I had known nothing about it. Ordinarily, as I've mentioned before, when the therapy is focused on sexual dysfunction, I want to see the other partner in the relationship, as well as the patient himself, and I want to talk with the two of them, both together and separately. In this case, however, my main objective was trying to deal with Doug's depression, and that had to take top priority, so I decided for the time being to delay bringing his wife into the picture.

Instead, I spent the next several sessions compiling as complete a psychiatric history and personality assessment of Doug as possible. As his story unfolded, it became increasingly bizarre—and more and more intriguing.

Doug had been married to his first wife, Lila, for more than eighteen years before her sudden death from a stroke at the age of forty-five. Yet in all that time, he had *never* had vaginal intercourse with this woman—not once in a period of nearly two decades. On an average of every four or five weeks, according to his recollection, he had obtained sexual gratification by dragging his penis back and forth between his wife's thighs. But he had never penetrated her vagina, and he was reasonably certain that no one else ever had, either. As far as Doug knew, Lila had been a virgin right up until the day she died.

He made it clear that this odd substitute for traditional intercourse had been totally his wife's idea. Beginning several months before they were married, he had attempted to have sex with her in the ordinary way, but she had steadfastly refused. She had also refused to engage in oral or anal intercourse, or even to manipulate his genitals with her hands. The only place she would allow his penis to touch her was between her thighs.

At first Doug had mistakenly believed that her refusal was based purely on moral or religious grounds. He thought that once they were married Lila would no longer have these reservations. But after the wedding, nothing changed.

"I just can't," she would repeat over and over again. "I just can't." It was the only explanation she ever offered.

By the time Doug revealed this situation to me, Lila had been deceased for four years, so there was no way of knowing what caused her to feel as she did or to be so adamant and uncompromising about it. Was she afraid of physical pain? Was she worried about getting pregnant? Was she a victim of incest or sexual abuse as a child and unable to overcome the memory of it? At this point, it was anybody's guess. Whatever her secret may have been, she had taken it with her to the grave, apparently without ever sharing it with anyone.

In spite of her weird behavior, Doug had cared deeply for Lila, and the suddenness of her loss came as a tremendous shock to him. It was a far greater blow, in fact, than he consciously realized at the time, and it set off a desperate search on his part for something to divert his attention, some way to regain at least a semblance of normalcy.

To many acquaintances and co-workers, his actions and attitude in the months immediately following Lila's death seemed callous and cold. He showed little if any outward grief. It was as though he wanted to forget that Lila had ever existed. He seemed to want to wipe away every trace of her presence in his life.

Doug gave all his late wife's clothes and personal possessions to charitable organizations. He got rid of all the household furnishings they had shared and had the place completely redecorated. He never bothered to buy a marker for her grave but spent thousands of dollars on a flashy new wardrobe for himself, and traded his conservative sedan for a sporty new convertible. He was often seen at exclusive restaurants and nightclubs, sometimes alone and sometimes with friends.

Soon he began dating a woman who had never been married and was fifteen years younger than he was. Her name was Lorraine, and she was a bank vice president who also happened to be a neighbor of Doug's. She lived less than a block away, and they had been casually acquainted for several years. Before long, they were spending several evenings together each week, although there was no sexual relationship, even after Lorraine started sporting an expensive diamond engagement ring.

To all outward appearances, Doug was a man in a terrific hurry to get on with his life and leave the past behind. Inside, however, he was in total torment, and his depression was deepening by the day. He had no appetite, and when he forced himself to eat, he often became ill. He was plagued by a variety of nagging aches and pains. He had difficulty going to sleep, and he had frequent bad dreams that jerked him awake suddenly in the middle of the night.

Doug convinced himself that getting married again would make things better, but he was wrong. He liked Lorraine, but in his depressed state he wasn't capable of really loving anyone. He felt no sexual desire for her, but he tried to have intercourse with her anyway. When he couldn't get an erection after several attempts, he seriously contemplated suicide, but he never quite got the nerve to go through with it.

Lorraine's reaction to Doug's impotency could best be described as sympathetic bewilderment. As incredible as it seems, his new wife was as much or more a stranger to sex as his first wife had been. In Lorraine's case, however, it was a matter of simple ignorance, not fear or revulsion. Although she wasn't unattractive, Lorraine had always been painfully shy, and outside her business environment, she still was. Until Doug came along, she'd never had more than a handful of dates, much less a steady boyfriend.

She knew next to nothing about sex, and, like Lila before her, Lorraine had never in her entire life experienced an orgasm.

Who says lightning never strikes twice in the same place?

Letting the Grief Out

Whenever anyone close to us dies, we humans must inevitably go through a grieving process. We have no choice in the matter. Different personalities have different ways of working through grief, but it's something that all of us have to do. For some, the process may involve weeping, wailing, and other dramatic outward displays of emotion. For others, it may require a period of solitude and quiet introspection. Still others resolve their grief by building some physical or symbolic memorial to the deceased or carrying out some task they believe would please the dead person.

Doug's problem was in trying to circumvent or ignore the grieving process. Part of the reason why he couldn't grieve normally was that he was uncertain of how he actually felt about Lila. On one level, his marriage to her represented nothing more than eighteen years of frustration and unresolved problems. But on another level, he surely cared about her in some way; otherwise he would have left her long before she died. Part of him was probably glad to be rid of her, and another part may have been angry at her for the freakish behavior she forced on him. But still another part of him remained stunned and saddened, perhaps even frightened, by her sudden loss.

In all likelihood, Doug had already been mildly depressed for a long time prior to Lila's death, but his inability to work through a mourning process for her sent his depression out of control and triggered all his myriad attendant problems, including his impotency.

Doug had been in therapy with me for several weeks when a seemingly minor incident finally allowed him to come to grips with his grief. He was driving to my office one morning to keep an appointment when he ran over a squirrel that darted in front of his convertible. It was one of those totally unavoidable things that happen thousands of times each day. Doug slammed on his brakes and swerved to miss the squirrel, but just as he did the animal reversed its course and went right under one of the front wheels of the car.

"One second it was running along, all graceful and full of life," he whispered hoarsely, "and the next second, it was lying there squashed in the street." Tears trickled down his face and onto the lapels of his jacket.

I was thinking that I'd never seen a grown man so utterly broken up about killing a squirrel when it dawned on me what was actually happening. It wasn't the squirrel that Doug was crying over—not at all. In reality, it was his unresolved hurt and anger over Lila's death that was now pouring out along with his tears.

After four years, Doug was finally mourning his dead wife. The squirrel was only the catalyst, the match that lit the fuse, as it were.

"I'm sorry you're upset," I told him quietly, "but I think you're very fortunate that that squirrel happened along when he did."

By the time he left my office that morning, the worst was over for Doug, although it took considerably longer for his grief resolution to run its full course. He visited Lila's grave several times, arranged to have an appropriate marker erected for her, and went through a series of emotional episodes. I encouraged him to talk openly about his conflicting feelings concerning his first wife, and he did. It was like removing a thorn from a festering, infected wound. He also continued to take an antidepressant drug for another two or three months, and by then he was doing much better.

In the meantime, I arranged to include Lorraine in our therapy sessions, and once she understood the background of Doug's depression and accompanying sexual difficulties, she was very supportive. This, in itself, was a major asset in Doug's recovery.

Today, more than two years later, I would classify Doug and Lorraine as a happily married couple with a normal, healthy sex life—and no need for Viagra. All things considered, I think that's quite an accomplishment.

Exploring the Unknown

In many respects, the human mind remains one of the "great unknowns" of modern science. Despite the vast knowledge gained over the past few decades about the inner workings of the human brain and the giant strides made in the field of psychotherapy, there is still much to learn.

We have, however, identified many distinct types of psychiatric problems that can profoundly affect sexual desire and/or performance, and medical science is in a better position to provide effective treatment than ever before.

But the day when swallowing a pill can effectively wipe out all the most common forms of mental illness, and the sexual problems that often go hand in hand with them, is still a long way off—if, indeed, it will ever come. In the meantime, psychotherapy, often combined with drug therapy, remains the most effective weapon in our arsenal for combating these disorders.

Let's take a brief look at some of the common psychiatric problems with sexual implications.

DEPRESSION—In the story of Doug, the reader saw some of the classic symptoms of the syndrome of depression. These include a sad, irritable, or depressed mood; loss of energy; difficulty concentrating; increased sensitivity; decreased appetite and weight loss; insomnia (although in atypical cases patients have increased appetite and oversleep); feelings of helplessness, worthlessness, and hopelessness; increased feelings of guilt; and thoughts of suicide or actual suicide attempts. As with Doug, patients aren't very interested in sex or anything else. They take no interest in themselves whatsoever or in the present or the future. Some depressions are so severe that patients have psychotic symptoms, such as hallucinations or delusions. They may hear voices and believe that people are plotting to hurt them. The more serious depressions are treated with a combination of antidepressant medications and psychotherapy. Practically all these medications can interfere with sexual functioning. Three exceptions are Wellbutrin, Serzone, and Desyrel. Desyrel (Trazodone) can cause priapism (persistent, painful erection). Since depression is a serious and potentially life-threatening illness, its treatment takes precedence over any concomitant sexual dysfunction. In the form of depression known as bipolar disorder (or manic depression), patients may actually become hypersexual during the manic phase of the illness.

ANXIETY DISORDERS—In these conditions, patients have apprehension or dread and what has been described as a sense of impending doom. Symptoms include a racing heart, palpitations, bandlike headaches, hyperventilation (rapid, shallow breathing), nausea, diarrhea, and increased urinary frequency. These disorders can take a chronic generalized form or occur in distinct episodes called panic attacks, which may be so severe that the patient is unable to leave home alone. Sometimes the patient is plagued with obsessive, recurrent, upsetting thoughts that he can't get out of his mind or by compulsive, repetitive acts that he thinks he must perform, such as a hand-washing ritual. Often so much energy is consumed with anxiety disorders that the patient has little interest in sex. One form of anxiety disorder is also classified as a sexual disorder. This is known as sexual aversion disorder, in which the patient has an extreme anxiety reaction to the point of revulsion when it comes to being touched or touching someone else sexually. In my experience, patients with sexual aversion disorder have suffered traumatic events such as rape or other forms of sexual abuse in childhood or adulthood. These conditions are, again, best treated by a combination of psychotherapy and anti-anxiety drug therapy. And, again, most anti-anxiety drugs can cause sexual dysfunction, although short-acting anti-anxiety medications can be used effectively if they are administered to the patient prior to sexual assignments.

ORGANIC BRAIN SYNDROMES—In these conditions, the very structure of the brain is affected. Patients with these disorders have difficulty with memory and orientation, typically being unable to remember the current date or their present location. Their emotional states can be very labile. They may suffer from hallucinations and delusions, and their intellect or judgment may be impaired, or they may have fluctuating levels of consciousness in delirium. Practically any serious medical condition, such as heart, lung, liver, or kidney failure, can produce these conditions. Fever, drugs, and alcohol use can also cause them. Other causes include strokes and degenerative conditions such as Alzheimer's, Parkinson's, and multiple sclerosis. Sexual desire is usually decreased in these conditions, but in some of the severe dementias the patient may become hypersexual. The physician's job is to first try to identify and treat the reversible kinds of organic brain syndrome, then to manage the chronic forms. All physicians should be alert to the fact that the first symptom a patient or partner may complain about is a decreased interest in sex.

SCHIZOPHRENIAS—These are a group of disorders characterized by the most unusual symptoms found in psychiatry: multiple auditory hallucinations directing the patient's thoughts and actions, an emotional tone that is often inappropriate to thought content (the patient laughs, for instance, while talking about the death of his father), thought disorders in the form of delusions of persecution or grandiosity, and thought patterns that are illogical and not goal directed. Conventional medical wisdom suggests that certain people are genetically predisposed to schizophrenic disorders, but environmental stresses often trigger the illness. Patients experience a living nightmare and have difficulty trusting others. Since true sexual intimacy requires a high level of trust, these patients have the most difficult time imaginable overcoming their feelings and allowing someone to get close to them. The best treatment consists of supportive psychotherapy, family education about the illness, and antipsychotic medication. I know I'm beginning to sound like a broken record, but the antipsychotic drugs—both old and new—can have an adverse effect on sexual desire and arousal, and some can interfere with orgasm.

PERSONALITY DISORDERS (BORDERLINE TYPE)—Patients with these personality disorders have very intense and unstable interpersonal relationships. They greatly fear abandonment and have a tendency to read signs of abandonment into the most innocent remarks or gestures by the partner. They have a great deal of difficulty controlling their anger, and it often becomes their most keenly experienced feeling. They have a shaky sense of self, tend to be impulsive, and may mutilate themselves or exhibit recurrent suicidal behavior. They are often depressed, although their depression isn't born of guilt but rather of boredom and emptiness. They often experience themselves as on the outside, looking in at others' relationships. Since their fear of desertion is so intense, they have difficulty maintaining a lasting, mature sexual relationship. I've seen patients with these disorders affected by every conceivable type of sexual dysfunction. The most effective treatment is in-depth individual psychotherapy, at times augmented by medication for such co-existing conditions as depression.

ALCOHOLISM—Although it's been mentioned in a previous chapter, I feel it would be remiss for me not to offer some additional comment on this very widespread disorder. Alcoholism is a major cause of erectile dysfunction, not to mention serious disruptions in families and relationships. All efforts must be directed toward getting the patient to stop drinking. Addressing accompanying sexual problems first by giving the patient a pill that helps him with erections while allowing his alcoholism to go unchecked makes no more sense to me than installing a big-screen TV in a house that's on fire.

10 Intrapsychic Factors

We've seen repeatedly in the past several chapters how sexual difficulties are often brought on by "mind over matter"—in other words, how purely psychological factors directly influence sexual arousal and performance. Although most of our case studies have focused on male problems, we've seen that women, too, can be adversely affected by these influences, and I've tried to show how psychotherapy can be used to overcome the problems.

But I've purposely saved the most difficult-to-understand psychogenic factor for last. None of the cause-and-effect relationships we've talked about so far is as hard to explain—or treat—as the ones we'll be examining in this chapter. In these intrapsychic factors, as they are called, the sexual dysfunction is a symptom of an unconscious internal conflict deeply rooted in the psyche. Tracking the conflict down and eliminating it so that the sexual dysfunction is relieved can be one of the most difficult tasks in psychiatry. It's usually a long, exhaustive process, both for the patient and the therapist.

In some of these cases, Viagra might make a positive contribution to the total treatment. In others, though, it might not help at all.

When an intrapsychic factor is involved, sexual acts and even the sex organs themselves take on strangely different meanings for the patient, who is usually aware of his sexual problems or inhibitions but totally unaware of their connection to the internal conflict that causes them. Through intensive therapy, the conflict can usually be traced to some early childhood crisis or trauma that was never resolved. The meaning applied by the patient to sex and the genitals is related to that earlier time, but the patient has no conscious awareness of this relationship.

Let's look first at a relatively simple case of sexual dysfunction stemming from intrapsychic factors, then move on to more complex illustrations.

New Problem, Old Roots

Nathan K., an investment broker in his late forties, had lived in New York most of his adult life, and his wife was a native New Yorker. They had been in Dallas for only about a year after being transferred from his company's Manhattan office when he came to me complaining of a premature-ejaculation problem that had come on quite suddenly and then progressed to erectile dysfunction.

"I've been happily married to the same woman for over twenty years, and up until the past few months, our sex life was fine," he said. "Nothing like this ever happened to me before, and I just can't figure out what's going on."

The abrupt onset of Nathan's difficulty was unusual in itself. Most men who ejaculate prematurely begin doing so during their early sexual experiences and generally continue in pretty much the same pattern as they grow older. Premature ejaculation seldom shows up "out of the blue" in midlife, as it had in Nathan's case. This made me wonder immediately if his recent move halfway across the country could have something to do with it.

"You're a long way from home," I said. "Has adjusting to a new environment been very stressful for you or your wife?"

"Not for me," Nathan said. "I love it here. Unfortunately, I can't say the same for my wife. Patty's been really grumpy and down in the dumps lately. We used to live just twenty minutes from her parents, and she could see them whenever she wanted to. She misses that a lot, and she's got friends in New York that she misses, too. I keep telling her she can make new friends, but she just doesn't seem interested."

From his troubled comments, I picked up a major clue to Nathan's sexual dysfunction. Although it would still take extensive therapy to get to the source of the problem, I had at least found a starting point.

Getting Worse, Not Better

As it turned out, Nathan's initial description of his wife's unhappiness over the move was a gross understatement. The situation was far worse than Nathan had first indicated. Patty was so embittered at being uprooted and "dragged off to this godforsaken wasteland," as she put it, that she refused to see any good whatsoever in her new surroundings. From the weather to the Texas dialect to the foods available in the supermarkets to the quality of the local theater, she condemned everything as "primitive and stupid."

This uncompromising attitude caused Patty to become clinically depressed, and she focused much of her irrational anger on her husband. She berated him constantly, loudly blamed him for her mental anguish, and refused to listen to reason or be placated. For a time, she was so turned off toward Nathan that it seemed pointless for him even to attempt having sexual intercourse with her.

Meanwhile, despite her animosity and ceaseless complaints about Dallas not being New York, Nathan did everything possible to mollify his wife, and he was very supportive when she began medical treatment for her depression. After she began antidepressant drug therapy, her mood improved slightly, but when she and Nathan tried to have intercourse, he was unable to control his ejaculation. And to make matters worse, he soon began having trouble getting an erection.

"My problem's getting worse, not better," he complained to me. "Can't you prescribe something that might help?"

By this time, of course, Nathan—like everybody else in the

country—had heard and read numerous reports about Viagra. He was convinced the "potency pill" was exactly what he needed, and I couldn't blame him for wanting to try it. In fact, I was sure it would offer significant short-term help for his surface sexual problems. Nevertheless, I resisted, knowing that real, lasting relief for Nathan involved more than swallowing a pill.

"It may not be the easiest way," I said, "but if you'll bear with me, I'd like to continue the psychotherapy for a few more sessions to try to get at the true source of the problem. After that, we can take a look at other options."

With obvious reluctance, Nathan agreed. I appreciated his willingness to tough it out, especially when many other physicians would have written him a quick prescription for Viagra and sent him on his way. I had learned a lot by now about his personal history and psychological background—enough to sense that the true underlying cause of his dysfunction was buried somewhere deep in Nathan's distant past.

That's precisely where I found it.

An Angry Mother Image

Nathan had spent his early years in a small midwestern town, the oldest of three sons born to what seemed on the surface to be a fairly typical middle-class couple. Nathan's father was a quiet, mild-mannered sales clerk for a local department store, and his mother was a talented but temperamental musician who earned almost as much money as her husband by serving as a church organist and giving piano lessons in her home.

As far back as Nathan could remember, his mother had been a volatile personality prone to angry outbursts, while his father was the type of man often stereotyped in those days as a "henpecked husband." The mother frequently shouted at the father and berated him in front of the children for his lack of initiative and mediocre earnings, but she reserved her more violent behavior for Nathan and his younger brothers.

During Nathan's grammar school years, he could scarcely remember a day when the three boys didn't incur their mother's wrath. She seemed to fly into a rage without warning and hit the boys with a belt, a switch, or the back of a hairbrush for no discernible reason. Nathan and the others lived in constant terror and did their best to stay out of their mother's sight and hearing, hoping to avoid punishment.

"Several times, I turned to my father for help," Nathan said. "I begged him to do something to protect us from that crazy woman, but he never did. Instead of standing up to her himself, he'd just tell us we ought to be more understanding of her because she was so 'nervous and high-strung.' It was so disgusting and disappointing. My father was such a weak-kneed little nothing of a man. He was pathetic, and I swore I'd never be anything like him."

Nathan also swore that he'd never marry a woman who resembled his mother in any way, form, or fashion. And when he met Patty, he thought he had found someone as opposite from "dear old Mom" as anyone could get. Patty admired him boundlessly, praised him effusively, and boasted to her friends about how fortunate she was to have married him. She gladly deferred to his wishes in any small differences they had, and never hesitated to show how dependent she was on him, both physically and emotionally.

For well over nineteen years, Patty remained an almost worshipful wife, and Nathan was allowed to play the role of dominant, assertive husband to his heart's content. Then came the move to Texas, the deepening depression, and the ominous transformation in Patty's personality. Next came the irrational fury, the out-of-control temper, the bitter accusations—just like his mother.

Even though Nathan didn't consciously associate the present situation with the fear and loathing of the past, deep in his subconscious it was exactly as if Patty, the sweet, yielding wife he had always known, had vanished into thin air and "dear old Mom" had come back to take her place.

"Well, if that's the way she wants it, fine," he roared during one of our sessions, "but I'm damned if I'll kiss her ass and kowtow to her like my father did!"

Bringing Conflicts to Light

Because of her depression and the angry change in her attitude and demeanor, Patty had "become" Nathan's mother, at least in her husband's subconscious mind. In turn, Nathan felt himself being forced into the role of his weak, passive father. It was when he rebelled against accepting this role that his sexual problems began.

Some men, like Nathan, equate orgasm with losing control and being "overpowered" by the woman, or with being made passive and submissive to her. In their minds, they are giving up something of themselves to the woman whenever they have an orgasm with her. The more hostile and combative the woman is, the more intense the man's reaction.

Nathan's premature ejaculations were his way of maintaining a measure of control and avoiding an orgasm during penetration that would signify a kind of surrender to his wife/mother. As these same subconscious defense mechanisms became stronger, they prevented him from getting an erection in the first place—an even more conclusive way to avoid giving in and being overpowered.

Successfully treating this type of problem is often very difficult because the patient has to understand that the symptoms he suffers in the here-and-now are merely manifestations of negative conditioning that took place long ago and far away. Nathan, however, was an intelligent, perceptive man who loved his wife. When he was able to get in touch with his angry feelings, realize that they were actually directed toward his mother, and place them in the context of his early childhood experiences, he was also able to separate his wife mentally and emotionally from his mother and solve his sexual problem.

Continued therapy for both partners defused a situation that could have led to the permanent breakup of this marriage for reasons that neither partner might ever have recognized without the therapy. Nathan was able to be more available to his wife, both sexually and otherwise, and more supportive to her during her depression. And as her depression lifted, Patty gradually became more and more like her old self again.

Even her attitude about Dallas changed for the better. "If you look hard enough, there really *are* signs of civilized life here," she remarked wryly the last time I saw the couple. "I actually found a decent bagel shop the other day."

The "Oedipal Phase"

It isn't fair to blame all of Nathan's problems solely on a flawed mother-son relationship. In fact, if Nathan had experienced his father differently—that is, as an emotionally strong man who could understand his wife and respond to her in a constructive way while also protecting his boys and keeping them from feeling so helpless—Nathan might never have appeared in this book.

The truth is, all of the intrapsychic problems that cause or contribute to male sexual dysfunction evolve from early unresolved dilemmas related to the adults with whom we spend most of our time during childhood: our parents. A child goes through a period between the ages of about three and a half to five when he or she "falls in love" with the parent of the opposite sex and views the parent of the same sex as a rival. Freud referred to this period in a small boy's life as the "Oedipal phase," a name drawn from a character in a Greek play by Sophocles who, not knowing their identities, killed his father and had sex with his mother.

Modern analysts don't believe that most four-year-old boys really want to have sexual intercourse with their mothers. A four-year-old doesn't understand the "ins and outs" of intercourse (no pun intended). But he does want to share intimate experiences with his mother by being fed, bathed, cuddled, and tucked into bed by her, and he views his father as an obstacle to these happy, intimate times with her. At the same time, however, he also loves his father and realizes that he is no physical match for the old man. Eventually, he gives up the hope of really winning Mom and comes to identify more with Dad, consoling himself with the idea that although he can't have Mom, he can at least grow up to marry a girl just like her.

In the meantime, many factors come into play during this phase in a boy's life, and later on they can cause glitches in the man's mother-concept. In Nathan's case, there was a double problem—a mother who was hard to love because of her temper and a father who was hard to identify with because of his weakness, which Nathan despised. Severe psychological trauma associated with either parent can have disastrous repercussions in adult life. (I'll describe an extreme case of this type later in this chapter.)

Another common example of a faulty mother-concept is the man who has no trouble relating sexually to his wife until the couple's first child is conceived or born. At this point, as the wife takes on the connotation of motherhood in the husband's mind, he is no longer able to feel sexual attraction or arousal toward her. In becoming a mother, she has also become forbidden territory—off limits to sex.

A man who harbors subconscious guilt feelings relating to his Oedipal phase may be particularly likely to transfer those feelings to his wife when she becomes pregnant or gives birth. Whenever this happens, psychological sexual dysfunction is the typical result.

The Madonna/Prostitute Split

For a normal man, it's important to fuse a certain degree of assertiveness with sexual intimacy. But when the assertiveness is distorted into hostility or repressed by fear, it often means trouble.

Some men become serial rapists because of a flawed mother-concept. Their relentless hostility toward women may develop as a result of being abused or abandoned by their mothers as helpless children. They rape for revenge, and their victims serve as psychological substitutes for their mothers.

Other men, although they aren't likely to resort to rape, also associate hostility with sexuality. Instead of using their penises as weapons to inflict punishment on women, they become obsessed with deeper-level fears of hurting the woman when they have sex. Consequently, they suppress their natural assertiveness, sometimes finding it impossible even to have sexual intercourse with their regular partners.

A man who has these fears may defend against them by placing the woman he loves on a pedestal, idealizing her and treating her with the greatest possible respect and admiration. To him, she is an angel floating on a cloud, and his feelings resemble the most extreme sentiments on a mushy Valentine's Day card: "I worship you. I adore you. I want to lavish you with tokens of my undying love. I want to shield you from all vulgarities, sacrifice everything for you, protect you from every harm."

At the same time, however, he refuses to allow himself to hold any sexual feelings toward her—much less to have sexual intercourse with her. In his mind, this would only degrade and defile her. He considers her totally above sex.

Deep within his subconscious, this man is equating his wife with his mother. When (and if) they have a child, the equation becomes even more pervasive.

This is the so-called madonna/prostitute split. It happens when a man separates sexual intimacy from assertiveness and is unable to combine the two elements.

In order to be assertive in sex, this same man must hold a woman in contempt and not care if he hurts her. This is why many men of this type patronize prostitutes or prowl singles bars in search of casual partners. Only when they find a woman who seems to be "beneath" them—someone for whom they can feel total disdain—are they able to assert themselves sexually.

Castration Anxiety

Then there are men with an irreconcilable fear of being hurt themselves during sexual intercourse. Again because of unresolved conflicts relating to Oedipal childhood experiences with their parents, these men fear their penises will be physically damaged or their genitals torn off if they have sexual intercourse. This fear is what gave this particular intrapsychic condition the name commonly applied to it by psychotherapists: castration anxiety.

I've treated a number of patients suffering from castration anxiety, but none was more severely affected than Raymond A., a veteran firefighter who had never been able to get an erection in the presence of a woman in all his forty-four years.

From our initial session, it was totally obvious that Raymond's erectile difficulties had no organic basis whatsoever. Despite his long history of sexual failure and a diagnosis of impotency, the patient really *wasn't* impotent due to any physical factors. He had no trouble obtaining erections when he was alone, and he reported masturbating at least every two or three weeks. He also had normal morning erections. But whenever a woman was present, both his sexual desire and his ability to perform completely deserted him.

"There was a time when I thought I might be homosexual," he said, "but I'm sure now that's not true. I've never felt the slightest sexual interest in another man."

When we began delving into his background, it quickly became apparent where the trouble had started. But when an intrapsychic disorder hides far back in time and in the patient's subconscious, just knowing the source of the problem may not be enough. It still has to be removed or neutralized, and that's never easy. Sometimes it proves to be impossible.

A Childhood of Tragedy

This patient's childhood had been so unhappy and marred by tragedy that merely hearing about it was upsetting. Actually living through it must have been sheer hell for Raymond.

He was born to a poor family on a small cotton farm in the Deep South, where illness, destitution, and death were never very far away. When Raymond was only two, his father contracted tuberculosis and died within a few months. Although Raymond was too young at the time to retain even the vaguest memory of his father, he was left with a sense of loss and bewilderment.

His mother was the glue that held what was left of his small world together, and he clung to her desperately with all his strength. But not long after his fourth birthday, she, too, was diagnosed with TB. Raymond was told that she was very sick, too sick to take care of him anymore, too sick to do anything but lie in bed and cough.

"You must stay away from your mama," his aunt told him sternly. "Else you'll catch what she has and die, too."

"She ain't gonna die!" Raymond remembered screaming. "I won't let her die."

But despite all his screaming, weeping, and praying, she did die. She died when Raymond was just over four and a half years old and in the midst of his Oedipal phase. This was the critical time in his young life when his need to be close to his mother would never be more intense. Yet for the last six months of her illness, Raymond was never allowed to go near her. He couldn't kiss her or hug her or do anything else to show his affection and how much he loved her.

Raymond didn't understand what TB was. All he knew was what his harsh old aunt told him—that if he got close to his mother, something terrible would happen to him.

Then, on the day of his mother's funeral, as if to deny every dire warning she had drummed into his head for months, the aunt scooped Raymond up in her arms, took him to his mother's open casket, and held him within a few inches of the corpse.

"Kiss her good-bye, Raymond," she said. "It's the last chance you'll ever have."

Filled with unspeakable dread, he broke free of his aunt's grasp and ran blindly out of the church.

Fears That Never Fade

Later, all that terror and confusion would flood through Raymond again any time he found himself near a woman. He could still re-call how violently he trembled and how sick to his stomach it made him when his sixth-grade teacher put her plump arm around his shoulders and kissed his cheek while congratulating him for earn-ing an A on a spelling test. The touch of her flesh against his had made his skin crawl, and the smell of her perfume seemed to be suf-focating him.

In high school, he went out on a few dates, but whereas other teenage boys were always looking for a chance to be alone with a girl, Raymond avoided these interludes at all costs. Once in a while he could stand to hold a girl's hand for a moment, but the thought of kissing her good night was more than he could bear. It always brought back the picture of his mother's dead face in her coffin.

This fear never faded for Raymond. Even after undergoing intensive psychotherapy and achieving a clear understanding of why he reacted the way he did, he remained terrified of being in an intimate male-female situation. To my knowledge, he was never able to get an erection with a woman, much less have sexual intercourse with one.

Raymond discontinued his treatments after a few months, and I eventually lost track of him when he moved to another city. The trauma of his childhood had created fears that were simply too deep and all-encompassing to erase. Even years of continuing therapy might not have allowed him to escape them.

I catch myself wondering sometimes if Raymond, wherever he may be, has had an opportunity to try Viagra—or if he would even want to. Frankly, I'm not convinced that the drug would do him much good, since it doesn't, in itself, stimulate sexual desire but only makes an erection possible in the presence of adequate stimulation. Could Viagra manage to slip past Raymond's fears long enough for a woman to get him sexually aroused?

At this point, I don't know. If, however, I ever encounter another patient with an intrapsychic problem as crippling as Raymond's but who is willing to persevere, I certainly look forward to finding out.

We can draw several fundamental conclusions from the stories of Nathan and Raymond. Among them are lessons that can benefit readers whose problems are far less demoralizing and destructive. They include:

1. Because we depend so heavily on our parents for such a long time, and because our basic psychological needs often relate back to them, we're all vulnerable to distorted

early images and emotions that can lead to intrapsychic disturbances.

2. Not all intrapsychic problems result in sexual dysfunctions.

3. Sexual dysfunctions that result from intrapsychic factors usually manifest themselves as sexual inhibitions, sexual anxiety, or problems in some phase of the sexual response.

4. When intrapsychic problems appear, they seem to come out of the blue without rhyme or reason, and the person experiencing them is unaware of the unconscious conflict.

5. These problems are best treated by a mental-health professional who has had training in in-depth forms of psychotherapy, such as psychoanalysis.

6. If a physician gives Viagra to an impotent patient with an intrapsychic problem, the underlying trouble remains untreated. All the physician has to show for his efforts is a patient with an intrapsychic problem and an erection.

11
Other Impotency Treatments

The effectiveness of Viagra and other new oral agents in relieving sexual dysfunction will lessen—but not eliminate—the need for other, less desirable impotency treatments.

Roughly 20 percent of all cases of erectile dysfunction, and almost half of patients with diabetes or prostate cancer, have failed to respond to Viagra. Other oral agents soon to be approved by the FDA may help in some cases where Viagra failed, but there will still be many men who require other measures.

It would be a mistake, then, to assume that the new oral agents have made all other approaches totally obsolete. Most men with erectile dysfunction will never again have to worry about needles, pumps, or implants, but for an irreducible minority of patients, these remain options that will have to be considered.

If Viagra doesn't work for you, however, your first choice as a possible alternative will probably be one of the other painless, convenient pills now under development. Let's take a look at them first.

Viagra's Competition

Test results reported with other new oral agents soon to be competing with Viagra have generally been less impressive than results obtained with Viagra itself. But this doesn't mean that these drugs can't help some patients with whom Viagra has been ineffective.

Two new pills for impotency are currently undergoing advanced clinical trials and are expected to be approved by the FDA. Little information has yet been released to the health care community on these drugs, and I've had no experience with them. While neither may measure up to Viagra in effectiveness, they still may help a sizable percentage of men with mild sexual problems.

One of these is an oral version of a drug called phentolamine, which has been used extensively in the past for penile injections. It works by gently dilating blood vessels in the penis, decreasing the viscosity of the blood, and blocking the effects of adrenaline. Developed by Zonagen, the drug is expected to gain final approval from the FDA sometime in 1998 and will be marketed under the trade name Vasomax. Thus far, studies suggest that only about 40 percent of users benefit from the drug.

The second is apomorphine, a nonnarcotic relative of morphine now being tested by TAP Holdings, which plans to market it as Spontane. The drug acts by stimulating the centers of the brain involved in producing an erection. In preliminary studies, 70 percent of mildly dysfunctional men found it useful, but it has no proven record of efficacy in cases of severe impotency.

Older Oral Agents

The search for an effective oral agent to relieve impotency has been going on for thousands of years. Various substances have been tried by countless millions of men all over the world, but unfortunately, until Viagra, no oral impotency drug has produced significant results.

Among the most widely used older drugs is yohimbine, a substance derived from the bark of the African yohimbé tree and the roots of a Southeast Asian shrub called rauwolfia. Available by pre-scription under two different brand names, Yohimex and Yocon, it is also sold in some states as an over-the-counter product.

Many claims have been made for yohimbine as an aphrodisiac and mood stimulator, and it may intensify sexual response in men with normal sexual function. But in the few small double-blind, placebo-controlled trials conducted with it, its success rate versus a placebo in overcoming erectile dysfunction has been spotty and modest at best. Many therapists have little regard for its efficacy, and the American Urological Association classifies it as "unproven."

When sexual performance problems are organic in nature, yohimbine appears to provide no appreciable help, but I've had some positive results with patients whose problems were psycho-logical. Patients with no identifiable medical cause for their sexual dysfunction sometimes report that it helps. Expecting too much from yohimbine is a mistake, but an increase in erectile function of 30 percent or so is significant for many patients, and I've seen the drug accomplish that. Just how much of this improvement resulted from the well-known "placebo effect" is, of course, impossible to determine.

My experience shows that, to be effective, yohimbine should be taken three times a day in carefully measured doses. This is why I always recommend the prescription version rather than over-the-counter products, which can vary widely in strength and quality.

Yohimbine's side effects include tremulousness, nervousness, ir-ritability, insomnia, headache, palpitations, minor elevations in blood pressure, and gastric disturbances, but only a small percent-age of users experience these symptoms. It can be dangerous to pa-tients with kidney disease or high blood pressure, and its labels also carry a warning about its use in older patients, those with diag-nosed psychiatric conditions, or persons with a history of gastric or duodenal ulcers.

Patients on antidepressants or mood-altering drugs are advised in product labeling not to use yohimbine. Ironically, some studies show it to be more effective when used in combination with an an-tidepressant called trazodone than when taken alone.

Trazodone has been around for years, but it remains something of an unknown quantity where impotency treatment is concerned. Researchers first showed interest in it as an erectile-dysfunction drug after some patients experienced priapism while taking it.

The risk of priapism alone is enough to persuade me never to prescribe trazodone in high doses. This ugly, painful condition can cause an attempt at sexual intercourse to end in a hospital emergency room, where surgery or injections to restore outward blood flow from the penis may be necessary.

I expect trazodone to remain in limited use as an antidepressant, but I certainly don't see it ever rivaling Viagra as a potency drug. Yohimbine may now retreat into the misty regions of folk medicine from whence it came, but some men may continue to buy it for its alleged properties as an aphrodisiac.

Other concoctions made from plants, insects, and animal parts have been used in many cultures in an effort to stimulate sexual desire and performance. Ancient man's first inkling that ginseng and fennel root held some sort of sexual powers may relate to the fact that both are shaped somewhat like an erect penis.

There are many examples of this kind of symbolism. In the Middle Ages, mandrake root, which resembles the human body, was worn around the waist as an amulet in the belief that it would cure impotence. Countless rhinoceroses have been killed by African natives who hoped that swallowing powder made from the ground-up horns of these mighty beasts would give their penises the strength and erectness of the rhino's horn.

Spanish fly is a legendary aphrodisiac derived from small beetles commonly found in France and Spain that contain a chemical called cantharidin. Whether Spanish fly actually stimulates sexual desire is still open to debate, but it is known that cantharidin is a powerful irritant. As it passes through the urine into the bladder and urethra, the chemical may have some stimulating effect, but it can also cause convulsions and, in extreme cases, death. Its outlawed status in the United States is fully justified.

Despite their persistent use all over the world, there is little scientific evidence that dietary and herbal remedies do anything to correct erectile dysfunction. Like the modern notion that eating oysters improves virility, most have little objective data to support the claims made for them. An exception may be Korean red ginseng, which has shown some promising test results, including increased penile rigidity and girth, longer duration of erections, and enhanced libido. The active ingredient in red ginseng is believed to be saponin, a soapy material found in many plants and used in various medications.

The Role of Testosterone

I know of a man in his mid-sixties who insists on having monthly testosterone injections in the belief that these shots will give him the sex drive and erections of a man half his age. This individual is outspokenly proud of the fact that he continues to have sex at least three or four times a week.

Testosterone injections may, indeed, help boost this man's libido, but I think he's kidding himself about them giving him better erections. Twenty-five years ago, many medical experts thought that low levels of testosterone were a major cause of erectile dysfunction, particularly in older patients. But later research shows no correlation between testosterone and erectile quality.

Testosterone is the primary male sex hormone—the masculine counterpart of the female hormone estrogen—and there are widely divergent views about the relative safety of artificially replacing testosterone in the body. Like the levels of estrogen in women, men's testosterone levels decline with age, and this is associated with a diminishing sex drive in older men, but not with inability to obtain erections.

Prior to menopause, the high levels of estrogen produced naturally in the female body help hold down a woman's risk of heart disease. Research indicates that after menopause, when estrogen levels decline sharply, hormone-replacement therapy may provide a woman with a measure of protection against heart attack and stroke. But no such benefits are attributed to testosterone—or to its replacement in men. In fact, some medical authorities warn that artificially boosting testosterone levels could increase the risk of some diseases.

Still, if a man's testosterone levels are extremely low, his interest in sex may become so nonexistent that getting an erection is virtually impossible. In this case, testosterone might help in ways that Viagra can't.

Testosterone injections can increase the sex drive in men with abnormally low natural levels of the hormone. Testosterone is also available in pill form, but in my experience the pills are relatively ineffective. For men whose testosterone levels fall into the normal range, administering it artificially has no effect on erections and can increase the risk of prostate cancer. Testosterone can also have the added liability of stimulating a man's sexual desire without doing anything to improve his performance.

Pumps and Needles

When erectile dysfunction stems from a purely physical cause, a patient's options are often far more limited than when the cause is psychological or a mix of physical and psychological factors. In studies, fewer than half the men who had undergone radical prostatectomies (removal of the entire prostate gland and surrounding tissue) were able to perform sexually even after taking Viagra. Patients with diabetes had a success rate of slightly more than half.

For such men, penile injections and vacuum pumps—as awkward and distasteful as they may be—may continue to be the only ways to get a predictable erection and perform sexually.

These devices *do* produce a reliable erection and one that works, at least in a mechanical sense. But they require a significant interruption in lovemaking, which can effectively "break the spell" for the man's partner and which is a primary reason why many of my patients who tried them never got around to using them with their partners. They can also cause considerable pain and discomfort.

The pumps, called vacuum constriction devices, or VCDs, consist of a plastic cylinder, a vacuum pump (usually connected to the cylinder by a tube), and an elastic constriction band. The cylinder, with the constriction band mounted on the open end, is placed over the penis. Air is then pumped out of the cylinder to create a vacuum, which, in turn, causes an erection. The constriction band is then transferred from the cylinder to the base of the erect penis to prevent the outflow of blood and maintain the erection, and the cylinder is removed.

The constriction band can be left on the penis safely for only about half an hour, and even in that period it can cause bruising and other discomforts. Some men also have difficulty operating the pump, which has to create the proper amount of negative vacuum pressure to obtain the desired effect. Battery-powered pumps are available for men who lack the strength or mechanical ability to operate a hand pump. For safety, only prescription models of these devices should be used.

The vacuum process takes a minimum of about six minutes to produce enough rigidity in the penis for vaginal penetration. Some manufacturers suggest pumping for a minute or two, then releasing pressure, then pumping again for three to four minutes, rather than pumping nonstop.

Besides the disadvantages already mentioned, the erections obtained with VCDs are far from natural, both in the way they feel and the way they act. The penis never achieves as much uplift as it does in natural erections, and its angle to the body isn't the same. The constriction ring also reduces blood flow far more than during a natural erection. It lowers the skin temperature of the penis, increases penile circumference, and causes the veins to be distended.

The pumps can also cause a problem known as "hingeing." Since the penis is often not as rigid as it would be in a normal erection, the man may have difficulty directing it where he wants it to go. This is not only awkward, but may actually cause injury to the penis during thrusting.

All told, it's no wonder that many men quit using VCDs after a short time. Yet many urologists continue to recommend them for their patients whose impotency is caused by physical factors.

Intracavernosal-injection therapy is another impotency treatment recommended by the American Urological Association. It involves injecting prostaglandin E (also known as alprostadil), a smooth-muscle relaxant marketed under the trade names Caverject and Edex, into one of the two corpora cavernosa in the body of the penis. Blood and pharmacologic agents easily cross over into the other corpora cavernosa, so that both sides of the penis are affected.

After the injection, it takes from five to twenty minutes for an erection to occur, meaning a potentially even longer delay in initiating intercourse than with a pump. This, again, causes widespread dissatisfaction among the partners of men who use injections because of the interruption and lack of spontaneity.

In close to 90 percent of the patients who use this therapy, erections are rigid, reliable, and last for at least an hour. On the negative side, however, they sometimes become "prolonged erections," which may not end for four to six hours. Beyond six hours, the ongoing erection is classified as priapism.

Both prolonged erection and priapism can inflict serious, irreversible damage to the smooth muscle tissue of the penis because of lack of oxygen. Patients whose erectile dysfunction is attributable to psychological or neurological causes are often more sensitive to the agents in penile injections, and their risk of prolonged erection and priapism is significantly increased. This is one major reason why an accurate diagnosis of the underlying cause(s) of impotency is so important.

Men who use penile injections for extended periods also complain of pains in the penis—usually a dull, aching sensation unrelated to the penetration of the needle itself. Some also report the formation of nodules at the site of repeated injections.

Intraurethral Suppositories

Next to Viagra, the newest type of impotency therapy is the intraurethral suppository, which utilizes alprostadil, the same drug used for penile injections, in a somewhat different manner. As of

1998, the only intraurethral suppositories available by prescription are those marketed by Vivus, Inc., under the trade name Muse. The name derives from "medicated urethral system for erection." At least one other company, Harvard Scientific Corporation, is currently developing and testing a similar product.

The main advantage offered by suppositories over injections is that instead of having to plunge a needle directly into the penis, the patient inserts an alprostadil pellet into his urethra (the normal pathway for urine) with a special applicator. The main disadvantages are that (1) the suppositories are generally somewhat less efficient than injections in producing erections, and (2) they impose certain restrictions on the man's activity while they take effect. The penis must be massaged for about ten seconds while the pellet dissolves, and some men have problems operating the applicators. In addition, the suppositories entail a distinct risk of priapism and prolonged erections, although not as high as with injections. Like the needles, suppositories also interrupt the normal lovemaking routine, sometimes for an even longer period.

Users are warned that lying down, especially on the back, during the first ten minutes or so after the pellet has been inserted will reduce blood flow to the penis and may impair the erection. Instead, men are advised to sit, stand, or walk during this period, which is hardly conducive to sexual activity. They are also told not to expect a normal-feeling erection, but one that may include mild pain or aching in the penis and/or groin and that may continue after orgasm. Even after the erection is over, the penis may feel full, warm, and sensitive to the touch.

Although intraurethral therapy produces a less consistent rigidity in the penis than injections, it has demonstrated its effectiveness in clinical trials in patients with severe impotency associated with cardiovascular disease, diabetes, postsurgical trauma, or pelvis injury, as well as with psychological causes. Overall, a little less than two-thirds of some fifteen hundred patients treated with Muse in one clinical trial achieved erections sufficient for intercourse.

Prosthesis Implantation

Implants of penile prostheses have been used to treat severe erectile dysfunction since the early 1970s. The earliest models consisted basically of two simple plastic rods surgically implanted in the penis. They gave the user what might be termed a "perpetual" erection.

But over the past twenty years, there have been many refinements and variations in penile implants. Failure rates due to mechanical breakdowns have been greatly reduced, and today's devices are generally very dependable. They fall into two basic categories: semirigid or malleable prostheses and inflatable (hydraulic) implants with one, two, or three components.

The semirigid and malleable versions seldom fail mechanically and require no manipulation before use; they are simply *there*. Whether flaccid or erect, the length and girth of the penis remain the same. Because of their flexibility, the malleable prostheses are easier to conceal than the semirigid ones. By contrast, patients need some manual dexterity to use the newer inflatable devices, but their big advantage is a more natural-looking penis, both in the flaccid and the erect states.

In my opinion, some of the hydraulic devices have gotten too sophisticated and the possibility of mechanical problems detracts from their practicality. If an implant fails, another surgical procedure is necessary to repair it, and if a man decides he no longer wants to have plastic rods or other mechanisms in his penis, they can only be removed surgically. Even the initial operation to implant the prosthesis causes such serious damage to the tissues of the penis that the user will never again be able to achieve a normal erection. There is also the possibility of infection whenever any foreign object is implanted in the body.

Despite these negatives, some men may still elect to go ahead with a penile implant. These devices are also endorsed by the American Urological Association, and for severely impotent men who don't respond to oral drugs and who find pumps, injections, and suppositories unworkable, they may represent the only solution to the problem. But the decision to have a prosthesis implanted should never be made in haste. Once the surgical procedure is done, it's difficult for the patient to change his mind.

In all likelihood, pumps, injections, suppositories, and implants will remain in limited use, but the days when they were hailed as great scientific breakthroughs against impotency are gone forever.

From your own standpoint, what's important here?

First of all, in spite of all the great things you've heard about it, Viagra may not be the drug for you. Maybe you tried it and got a splitting headache. Perhaps you're on a medication that contains nitrates and the combination could pose serious health risks. Maybe you have a retinal disease, and your opthalmologist cautioned you not to use Viagra. Or maybe you took the new drug and it simply didn't work for you.

Will the next generation of oral agents have different or fewer side effects? Will you be able to take them with nitrates? Will they affect some people's vision? We won't know until all the studies are in, but they may offer viable alternatives to Viagra.

As passé as it may seem to keep taking yohimbine with Viagra readily available, I have patients who have been helped by yohimbine, learned to rely on it, and have no intention of switching to anything else.

Although inconvenient, mechanical procedures such as injections may be more effective in men with the most severe types of organic erectile dysfunction from prostatectomy or diabetes. Your urologist can advise you about the best approach for your individual needs.

12
Winners, Losers, and "Super Sex"

Most sports fans are familiar with one of the oldest truisms of sporting competition, one summed up in a philosophical observation by Grantland Rice, the famed sports columnist of the 1920s: It matters not who won or lost, but how you played the game.

It was, and is, a noble thought. Unfortunately, nothing could be much further from the truth today, either in American sports or American society in general. Some people still give lip service to the idea that graceful, valiant losers deserve as much respect in defeat as exultant winners do in victory. In reality, though, things usually don't work that way anymore. We idolize the batter who hits the most home runs and disregard the player who merely bunts well. We worship the running back who scores the most touchdowns and ignore the blockers who clear a path for him. We shower the champion with limitless adulation and forget the runner-up who fell an inch or a point short.

Over the years, most of us have heard countless members of highly successful professional football teams express the same basic sentiment as they prepare for the Super Bowl. It goes something like this: "It doesn't make any difference how many times you win during the regular season and the play-offs. If you get to the Super

Bowl and lose, none of the rest matters. Losing here is the worst thing that can ever happen to you. It eats away at you all during the off-season."

If a single loss, after reaching the pinnacle of their profession, represents nothing more than the "worst thing that can ever happen" to these players, then I can only feel sorry for them. This selfish, negative attitude is about as far as you can get from Grantland Rice's philosophy, and yet this is what all of us are conditioned to believe nowadays. It's part and parcel of our national "win or else" mentality.

Is it any wonder, then, that sexual failure—either real or imagined—after a lifetime of relative success and fulfillment can become the humiliating focal point of a man's entire existence?

Mr. Average Versus Mr. Wonderful

Winning (and being able to classify ourselves as winners) at any cost has become an obsession—not merely in athletic contests but in all aspects of life. Under the competitive, dog-eat-dog game plan of the 1990s, there is little regard for also-rans and second-bests, and nothing but disdain for those identified as losers. Regardless of how disreputably he may have achieved his success, the "top dog" is inevitably the person who commands admiration and envy. Everyone else is inferior.

For an incredibly large number of men and women, this harsh, unforgiving philosophy takes control of their most important relationships, both professional and personal. When it does, even making love can become a game of winners and losers.

In such an environment, being cast as an "ordinary guy"—especially in a sexual sense—can be a disturbing, even demeaning experience. It can lead to nagging inner doubts and questions. "Average sex" may be perfectly good sex, but let's face it, it's not "super sex," either. Does that mean a lot of other guys are better at it? Is "average sex" as meaningless to some women as "those other" football games are to a Super Bowl player? And even at his best, is an "ordinary guy" actually capable of "super sex"?

Many men fight an endless battle to keep from being tagged as "Mr. Average" and to portray themselves as winners in at least some aspect of life. This helps explain why a mild-mannered clerk who spends his days stuck in a menial, dead-end job may suddenly turn into a raging "road warrior" when he climbs behind the steering wheel of his car on the way home.

"I may not do too well at work," his subconscious is trying to tell us, "but I'm still the best driver with the hottest car on the freeway, so the rest of you losers better watch out!"

Likewise, the weekend athlete who never seems to win at golf or tennis can compensate by thinking of himself as a champion lover in his own bedroom. The man who knows deep inside that his life will always be a financial struggle can console himself with the idea that he is still a hero to his wife and children.

We know what frequently happens to "road warriors." They often end up killing themselves or someone else with their automobiles. Often less obvious—but just as tragic in its own way—is what can happen to the self-styled "hero" or "great lover" who suddenly has that distinction rudely torn away, leaving him exposed as just another "ordinary guy."

In a world without sympathy for losers, he simply may not be able to forgive himself for turning into one, at least in his own mind. And he may find himself impotent as a result—which can only reinforce his loser image.

From Impatient to Impotent

The unhappy experience of Howard K. provides a case in point.

Howard's favorite slogan was "You have to spend money to make money." He repeated it over and over every day. With Howard, though, the problem was that he kept spending money he didn't have, then hoping against hope to recoup his expenditures.

For nearly five years, Howard managed to maintain an opulent lifestyle for himself, his wife, Carla, and their two children, despite the fact that the small construction company he owned was in deep financial trouble. The company, which Howard had started on a shoestring when he was twenty-eight, had always provided a decent living for the family, but by the time he turned thirty-five, Howard was no longer satisfied with that.

He was impatient with the small victories of the past. They had grown meaningless for him, and he had visions of much grander triumphs.

Howard, you might say, was ready for the Super Bowl.

His first key mistake was assuming an oversized mortgage on a large house in an exclusive development, then borrowing money to fill it with luxurious furnishings. Howard thought these showy trappings would help him land construction contracts with many of the wealthy people who were buying lots in the development. To impress prospective clients, Howard also insisted on maintaining a costly country club membership, entertaining lavishly, and driving a forty-five-thousand-dollar BMW.

Within a year or two, Howard's monthly obligations climbed to about three thousand dollars a month more than his income from the company. His solution was to borrow more money.

As his financial situation grew increasingly desperate, Howard began the ruinous practice of using the money from down payments received on construction jobs to pay his personal debts, thus leaving him with no funds to buy materials to complete the jobs. Soon, all his credit cards were maxed out, and the banks refused to extend him further credit.

To make matters worse, Howard concealed the situation from Carla for as long as he could. Carla was an experienced real estate broker, and when she finally discovered how far in debt they were, she told Howard repeatedly that she wanted to go back to work to help get them out of the hole they were in. But Howard adamantly refused to hear of it.

"I can take care of this family," he stormed. "You just stay home with the kids, and let me worry about the business. Everything will be fine."

It wasn't, of course. Eventually, Howard was forced to declare bankruptcy. He lost his company, the big house, and all the furnishings. The BMW was replaced by an eight-year-old Toyota, and the family moved into a rented duplex. Howard took a modest job as a sales representative for a building-materials supplier, and Carla returned to the real estate business, where she quickly began earning almost twice as much as Howard.

It was about six months after his bankruptcy when Howard made his first visit to my office. He wasn't quite forty years old, and he was totally impotent.

"Up until I went broke, I'd never had any sexual problems in my whole life," he said, shaking his head. "The urologist says there's nothing wrong physically, but I can't do a damned thing. I feel like such a failure."

"Have you talked to your wife about the problem?" I asked.

"Not really," he said. "I've just been avoiding it, to tell the truth. I appreciate the way Carla helped bail us out when I lost everything, but I guess I feel kind of bitter, too. She really put me down hard when she found out what a mess we were in. Made me feel like a total washout."

After meeting with both Howard and Carla, I was soon able to get a fix on Howard's problem—although "fixing" Howard himself wasn't quite so simple. Because she had taken control of the family finances and was earning a better salary than he was, Howard now saw Carla as a competitor instead of a partner. In his mind, she had emerged as the winner in the situation and he was left as the loser. His impotency was directly related to these feelings of resentment and anger.

Another physician prescribed Viagra for Howard, but it didn't immediately produce the desired results. The first time Howard took a pill, he got an impressive erection within an hour. But he said nothing to Carla about taking the drug, and when he went into the bedroom, primed to make love for the first time in half a year, he found her sound asleep. The second time he tried it, he again failed to tell her beforehand, and she put him off, claiming she had a headache.

It was only after I saw Howard in individual psychotherapy that matters started to improve. I learned that he had always had feelings of inadequacy. As an adolescent, he was smaller than the other boys and suffered from severe acne, both of which affected his self-image. His father, a former Marine who had been highly decorated for valor in World War II, was very critical of Howard, and his regular belittling aggravated Howard's problem.

Howard attended a large state university but failed several major courses of the type that, according to Howard, "separated the men from the boys." He dropped out of school and joined the military, but he was too depressed to make it through basic training and received a medical discharge, then had to come home in humiliation to face his disgusted father.

Howard's life became a repetitious pattern of defeat. An uncle hired him in a family business, and at first he did a good job. But then he was assigned to open and head a new branch office, and the responsibilities seemed too great for him to cope with, so he failed again. It was clear from his story that each time Howard approached success, he sabotaged himself and arranged to fail, thereby reinforcing his feelings of worthlessness and his belief that his father would always be the winner and he the loser.

The breakthrough came when Howard realized that there didn't have to be one winner and one loser in a situation. Instead, he and his father could both be winners—and he and Carla could both be winners, too. Once he understood this, he and his wife could also be lovers again.

Carla helped by assuring Howard that she cared deeply about him and that she hadn't purposely tried to displace him as the family breadwinner. "I don't care about making piles of money," she said. "All I want is for everything to be back like it was before all this happened."

As it turned out, Howard's sexual function came back without the use of Viagra. "Our sex life has never been better," he told me a few weeks later. "Everything's super." Not the same kind of "super" as in the Super Bowl, I thought, but a lot healthier and more realistic.

Here are some thoughts to consider in Howard's case:

1. Howard had an apparent need to excel and always do better, but his actions belied that need and pointed to a deeper problem.
2. Howard habitually undercut himself by sabotaging his own successes.
3. Although he was outwardly aware of his need to win, Howard was inwardly unaware of his need to defeat himself.
4. Howard's defeats protected him from facing the anxiety connected with his unacceptably aggressive wishes directed against his own father.
5. Howard's erectile dysfunction was a ticket into my office that eventually enabled him to settle these complex internal conflicts through psychotherapy.
6. Just giving Howard a pill to improve his erections would have accomplished little in the long run, and Howard would still have been just as big a loser, even with an erection.

If you see something of Howard lurking in yourself, you aren't unusual, but you probably also aren't a good candidate for Viagra.

Wanting More, More, More!

One way in which many of us try to confirm our status as winners is by constantly reaching out, like Howard, for bigger and better things—a more expensive car, a house in a "better" neighborhood, a more extravagant vacation than the one we took last year, a loftier position on the corporate ladder, and so forth.

To paraphrase a popular soft-drink commercial, we want more, more, more! And only as long as we get it can we sustain our identity as winners. But when men try to apply this concept to their sexual experiences, trouble and disappointment are usually the result.

I'll never forget the chagrin and distress of a woman patient in her mid-thirties who came to me for therapy several years ago.

"I'm afraid I may be frigid," she said uneasily. "At least that's what my husband says. He's upset because he doesn't think I get aroused as much as I should and I don't always have an orgasm when we make love."

After she gave me a detailed history of their relationship and her own background, I found that her desire and arousal phase were totally normal. She also told me that she was able to reach orgasm about 90 percent of the time while she and her husband were having intercourse. This was completely acceptable to her, she said, and she had no complaints about their sex life. It was her husband who was complaining and saying that something must be wrong.

Later, when she was able to persuade her husband to come in and talk to me, I discovered him to be a very husky, macho-type individual who seemed vain and obsessive about his sexual prowess. He simply couldn't understand why his wife wasn't swept away on wild flights of passion each and every time they had sex. He had tried to convince himself that his wife's "frigidity" was to blame, but in reality he was having doubts about his own performance.

"A real man should be able to make his wife have an orgasm one hundred percent of the time," he said. "And since there's no doubt that I'm a real man, there's got to be something wrong with her."

I did everything possible to reassure the woman. I also tried to explain to the husband that his wife was sexually normal in every respect, and that many factors could affect her orgasms, but I'm not sure if he ever understood—or if he really *wanted* to understand. I sympathized with the wife, but I also felt sorry for the man. God help him if he ever develops erectile dysfunction. He's the type of individual who could become suicidal if confronted by his own sexual failure.

The case above demonstrates a fairly common situation. The female partner is identified by the male partner as having a sexual problem, but this is actually the man's way of dealing with his own insecurities. He defends his own fragile sense of sexual adequacy by using a macho character style and projecting his sexual doubts onto his partner. In other words, "I'm not the one with a problem, you are. So go to a doctor and get yourself fixed."

But before a man jumps to this conclusion, it's a good idea for him to ask himself a few key questions: What's my responsibility in this unsatisfying sexual relationship? Might I have contributed to the problem? Are my sexual expectations realistic for my partner? Do I ever put her needs before mine? Do I put the entire responsibility for my sexual gratification on her?

If you answered "none," "no," "no," "no," and "yes," it's time to grow up and take the elevator to the adult floor.

Searching for Ms. Goodbar

The desire to prove oneself sexually beyond the confines of a committed relationship is an urge that many men feel at times. Some experience it only rarely or fleetingly, but for others it can become a constant, compulsive drive. Regardless of the circumstances, yielding to the urge is invariably fraught with many dangers: permanently broken relationships, divorces, abandoned children, unwanted pregnancies, AIDS and other sexually transmitted diseases, to name a few.

Ask a hundred different unfaithful men what caused their infidelity, and they may well list a hundred different reasons, none of which sounds exactly the same as any other:

"My wife doesn't understand me. All she does is nag."

"My wife's let herself go to pot. She doesn't care how she looks anymore."

"She's always tired or feeling bad, and she never seems interested."

"I was under heavy pressure at work, and my secretary was always there for me. I felt drawn to her emotionally, and one thing led to another."

"I love my wife, and I never meant for it to go this far. But when this foxy twenty-year-old started flirting with me, I just couldn't resist."

And so on.

Most of the time, however, at least in my experience, when a man strays from an established relationship, the real explanation is almost always the same: He is seldom willing to take even part of the responsibility for the problems, but he no longer feels content with his existing situation and wants something better. Something more.

He's bored and weary with average, ordinary sex, and his regular partner may seem to feel the same. She definitely doesn't turn him on the way she once did, but the worst part is that he obviously doesn't turn her on the way he once did, either. His ego starts to suffer, and so, in all likelihood, does his sexual performance.

With a nostalgic sense of loss, he recalls some of his earlier sexual adventures. Some of them were so good, so fulfilling, and some of the women were so sensual and adoring. They made fireworks go off and bells ring. They made him feel so strong and in control. Like he could actually fly if he wanted to. And they made him feel so loved and so lucky. Like a world beater. Like Superman.

So what happened? How did all that just vanish? How did making love change from life's ultimate thrill to just another weekly (or monthly or semimonthly) chore?

There has to be more to it than this, he thinks. There *has* to be.

Most of the time, he tries to tell himself it's *her* fault. But deep inside, he knows that isn't completely true. He's certainly lost something along the way, too, and the loss makes him feel diminished and uncertain. But under the right circumstances, he's pretty sure he could get it back again.

With the right person, he rationalizes, maybe he could rediscover "super sex."

When Adequate Isn't Enough

If what I've encountered in my thirty-plus years as a physician and sex therapist can be used as a guide, I think it's safe to say that many American women are unaware of how critical the "average guy" is of his own sexual performance.

Millions of men aren't satisfied with an "adequate" sexual experience. But they are conditioned to want more than they frequently get, not only out of the sex act itself but out of themselves as well—especially in such areas as size, rigidity, and duration of erections. Interruptions and distractions that cause them to lose focus often have direct negative effects on their erectile function.

Also, as paradoxical as it may seem, the more intensely a man wants sex, the more flawed his performance may be—at least by his own critical standards. As one man expressed it: "I can't believe how far behind I can get and how fast I can catch up." I think most men have an inherent understanding of what this statement means in a sexual context, but I suspect many women may be puzzled and confused by it.

The fact is, performance anxiety is often the sole cause of sexual dysfunction. It is also a contributing factor for a large percentage of the men who seek treatment for their problem.

Millions of women are sympathetic and concerned about the delicate interrelationship between their partner's ego and his sexual performance. Others, though, are less perceptive. When their partners fail, they are hurt and disappointed. They can also become angry at the man, particularly if they hold the erroneous belief that a man can control his erections. In such cases, the woman's reaction can make the problem worse.

There is some justification for the widely held opinion among women that a man's main interest is in the act itself, rather than the affection and emotional closeness on which women place a high value. Certainly, some men do have what could be described as a "wham bam, thank you, ma'am" approach to sex, but I've found that many others are just as sensitive to its larger implications as are their female counterparts. (I'll discuss the female sexual response in greater detail in a later chapter, along with possible benefits offered by Viagra to women.)

The fact remains that women don't have to be initially interested or desirous in order to participate in sex. Up to a point they can also fake arousal, while men can't, although without stimulation and actual arousal, a woman will not lubricate. Still, with artificial lubrication an unaroused woman can at least participate in intercourse. An unaroused man clearly cannot. Thus, the burden of performance rests squarely on the male, and when lovemaking is less than "super," men tend to feel responsible.

In the beginning of a relationship, especially when the couple is young, just lying nude next to his partner is often quite sufficient to get the man aroused and erect. But with age and accumulated sexual experience, the man will need more direct sexual stimulation. If his wife is not an enthusiastic partner and continues to remain passive, sexual problems will most likely occur. I believe it's extremely important for the woman to have as clear and broad an understanding as possible of her husband's sexual response. It's equally important, of course, for the man to understand his wife's response. This kind of mutual understanding is the surest way to eliminate unrealistic perceptions about "super sex."

Viagra has proved itself capable of solving the immediate problem of erectile dysfunction in the majority of men. For millions of men who are dissatisfied or insecure with their sexual performance, it can provide a tangible security blanket. But it can't create the loving, giving attitude that makes sex between two people genuinely special and satisfying.

As one of the guests on a recent edition of ABC's *Nightline* observed during a discussion about Viagra: "Erection isn't communication."

Morals and Medical Ethics

How far should the health care community go in allowing Viagra to be used as a convenient tool for obtaining better sex, rather than as a serious medicine for treating clinical sexual dysfunction? This question raises important ethical issues that all physicians now prescribing Viagra must confront on a daily basis.

From all indications, some of the overwhelming demand for Viagra is coming from normal, healthy men who merely wish to improve their sexual experiences and feel generally "sexier" and more confident about themselves. These men are among the hundreds of thousands who have deluged clinics and doctors' offices coast to coast asking for Viagra.

Many of them may have unbelievably high expectations about what the drug will do for them. But if every man in America should see Viagra as the answer to all his sexual fantasies—the opportunity to become the sexual Superman he's always dreamed of being—the drug could bring on a social and/or medical catastrophe.

As *Time* magazine noted in a May 1998 cover story on Viagra, "According to Pfizer, there's no evidence that overeager users could develop a physical addiction to Viagra. But as for a psychological addiction, that is uncharted territory."

As I've stressed before, Viagra has no aphrodisiac qualities, yet the very *idea* of it can cause erections in a sizable percentage of men. As one patient confided, "Most of the time I don't even need the pill. It's enough to know it's there in my pocket, just in case."

This, in itself, is an indication of psychological dependency, and many men with access to the drug may not be willing to run the risk of failure by trying to have sex without it.

One of the patients involved in the clinical trials of Viagra prior to its FDA approval admitted to downing one of the pills practically every night. "That way, if something happens when we get in bed, I'm ready to let nature take its course," he said. "If it doesn't, I just forget about it and go to sleep."

A *Newsweek* article tells of other cases of outright abuse and potential overuse of the drug: A seventy-seven-year-old man, obviously planning to make up for lost time, asked his doctor for one thousand pills at once (he actually ended up getting only thirty), and a Milwaukee urologist ran an ad on the Internet offering a telephone consultation and a Viagra prescription for fifty dollars. And *Time* mentioned two other men in their seventies, one of whom "turned into a monster" after taking the drug, who were planning to invite their friends to a "Viagra party."

Even among the elderly, it seems, the concept of "super sex" is alive and well.

Under certain conditions, I'm not opposed to prescribing Viagra for men with minimal loss of sexual function, but before I do, I want to know something about the individual patient and how he intends to use the drug. In my view, a physician's role is to dispense sound medical advice and proper treatment, not to make moral judgments. But at the same time, I would never conduct sex therapy with a couple if I knew that one (or both) of them was having an affair outside the relationship. And under no circumstances would I offer sex therapy to a man and his mistress or a woman and her extramarital partner.

My reasons for this are primarily legal rather than moral ones. If I were to prescribe Viagra for a man in these circumstances, I could expose myself to litigation by the spouse. It would be entirely possible for a husband or wife to sue me for enabling his or her mate to consummate an affair with another partner.

I'd be doing no one a favor, anyway, by prescribing Viagra for a man willing to forsake his mate in search of "super sex." If the promise of the drug should lead him to doomed expectations of unattainable sexual perfection, he might sue me, too.

The most important reason, however, for not treating a man or woman who is having an extramarital affair is that the cheating partner can't be expected to invest emotionally in therapy aimed at improving the marriage. From my standpoint, Viagra is simply another tool for effecting such improvement—albeit a very effective one—and it's only within this context that I'm willing to use it.

Doctors all over the country may have their principles—and their malpractice insurance—tested by such situations as the Viagra Revolution runs its course.

Staying in Sync Sexually

If a couple is genuinely willing to work at it—and if there is respect, caring, and affection on both sides—I think that "super sex" is every bit as possible between two partners who have been together for forty or fifty years as it is between a man and a woman who have just met.

In many instances, Viagra can play a vital role in this. But there's also another side to this story. Both parties have to be sexually in sync. Otherwise, Viagra can actually be hazardous to a relationship.

Many couples have established an unofficial status quo where sexual activity is concerned, and introducing Viagra can throw this out of balance. Suddenly, a man who has avoided sex for months or years becomes sexually demanding and eager to demonstrate his new virility and prowess several times a week. But his wife has learned to live with little or no sex over a sustained period, and she may not be prepared for or receptive to so much abrupt amorousness.

As *USA Today* writer Karen S. Peterson noted in a recent article on Viagra, "Couples who have taken each other—and impotence—for granted for years may need to learn new techniques. Others may have to look into motives as well as methods."

The story of Howard and Carla illustrates how ineffective Viagra can be if one partner tries to use it without the full knowledge and cooperation of the other.

Unless a mutually agreeable middle ground can be found, the marriage may suffer greater damage instead of undergoing repair. The woman may nervously withdraw even further, and the man may decide he wasted his money on those ten-dollar pills. And, of course, each may also turn away from an unresponsive mate and look for greener pastures elsewhere.

There's also another extreme to consider. A woman who feels sexually deprived may pressure her partner to get Viagra, and this can make him even more anxious and insecure about his sexuality. As much as a man may appreciate "sexiness" in a woman, he can be intimidated if her sexual desires and demands become too strong.

Used with common sense, discretion, and consideration for one's partner, Viagra can help unlock the door to a better sexual experience for men and women alike. It can be a win-win situation all the way around. But if sex is ever to be really "super," it must earn that rating from both partners.

13
How Often Is "Normal"?

Subtly related to many Americans' distorted notions about "super sex" is the pervasive idea that men and women are *supposed* to have sex a certain number of times each week or each month. If this were true, then it would naturally follow that those who fail to conform to this arbitrary number are somehow abnormal.

The point is, however, that it *isn't* true. As much as we like to impose quotas and standards on all types of human behavior, and although we read and hear a lot of speculation about how much sex we have to have to "keep up with the Joneses," sexuality remains a highly individual matter. What's too much for one person may not be enough for another, and vice versa.

Women, of course, have no physical limitations on the number of times they can have sex. Some female prostitutes have been known to have sex with dozens, even scores, of partners in a single night, a feat that no four or five men put together could hope to match. Thus, in terms of capacity, men are at a decided disadvantage, and this helps explain why the numbers game can assume such huge significance in the masculine mind.

Numbers sometimes become an ego thing, in which men compare their own performance with an average based on hearsay or a sex study published in some magazine. With certain men, failure to measure up numerically may be seen as a negative reflection of their manhood, and they may force themselves beyond their limits in an effort to make up the deficit and "prove" themselves. This is a factor in many cases of infidelity. Carried to extremes, it can also lead to performance anxiety and erectile dysfunction.

A Question of Variables

The claims of some professional athletes notwithstanding, only a small minority of men with especially strong sex drives and unlimited opportunity for sexual activity are likely to average having sex as frequently as once a day over a sustained period of time. This isn't to say, of course, that no man is capable of having multiple daily orgasms and/or sex partners, at least for a few days or a few weeks; some men undoubtedly are, but they are exceptions to the general rule. Men who are this active sexually are usually very young, very healthy, and not overly burdened with other activities and responsibilities that require a lot of time and energy.

A good example of such a man might be a recent bridegroom in his mid-twenties who is enjoying a prolonged honeymoon. Over a period of weeks, this young man and his wife may average making love, say, twice a day, possibly even more. But there's no reason for another man of the same approximate age and physical condition to try to match this feat, especially one who has been married for five years and works nine or ten hours a day.

There are many variables involved in determining what amount of sex is "right" for any given person. The age of the individual definitely plays a major role. So does the duration of his primary relationship—and whether, indeed, he has such a relationship. Other factors include how busy he is, how many distractions he faces, how much energy he has, the sexual needs of his partner, and, of course, his own "sexual clock."

There's certainly nothing abnormal about slowing our sexual pace as we grow older. In my experience, daily sex is usually reserved for the very young and robust, but there are certainly exceptions. I know of one wealthy man in his mid-sixties who still claims to have intercourse with his much younger girlfriend "at least once a day," and I'm aware of other men well up in their seventies who are still quite capable of frequent orgasms.

At any rate, because of all the variables involved, I actually prefer to avoid the term "normal" as it relates to the usual frequency of sex. It seems somewhat less discriminatory to talk in terms of averages.

If you could survey every twenty-five-year-old man in America on the question of how often he has intercourse, I think you might come up with an average answer of around two times per week. For all men of sixty-five, the average might be two times a month. But these are purely "ballpark" figures. The truth is, nobody really knows what is average, much less what is "normal."

People are different. We don't all wear yellow neckties. We don't all like chocolate mousse. We don't all drive Toyotas. And none of us has to be governed by someone else's norms where sex is concerned.

Considering Your Partner

How much sex is too little? How much sex is too much? There's no universal answer or "one size fits all" equation that answers these questions. To a great extent, it depends as much on the man's partner as it does on the man himself.

If a couple in a long-term committed relationship has sex only two or three times a year and is happy and content with that arrangement, there's absolutely no reason for them to think of themselves as freaks of nature, much less to be regarded as such by others. After all, fulfilling each other's physical and emotional needs is this couple's only responsibility. As long as they accomplish this to their mutual satisfaction, what they do and how often they do it is nobody else's business.

When problems do arise, they are commonly found in one or both of two major areas: (1) one partner's sexual needs and desires may be more intense and frequent that the other's, meaning that he or she wants to have intercourse considerably more often than the other; (2) the couple may have approximately the same level of sexual need but be out of sync as to when and where it's appropriate to have sex.

When one partner's sexual need is greater than the other's, some "give and take" and a caring, cooperative attitude usually offer the best hope for an equitable solution. A woman is physically capable of having sex more often than she might prefer, so if the woman is the less motivated partner, she may be willing to acquiesce to her mate's wishes, at least part of the time, in order to accommodate him. The man, meanwhile, must learn to "cool it" occasionally when he finds himself on a higher sexual frequency than his partner.

When the situation is reversed, however—that is, when the woman often finds herself in sexual "overdrive" while the man is stuck in "neutral"—it may be considerably more difficult to resolve. In this instance, a careless approach can make matters even worse, because a man pushed beyond his limits for arousal and performances is a likely candidate for sexual dysfunction. It's important to remember that if both the man and his partner agree, the couple can satisfy each other sexually in ways other than intercourse.

Today sexual equality is the norm. Sexually assertive women are commonplace, and as I've mentioned before, their assertiveness can be sufficiently unnerving to trigger performance anxiety in some men.

Viagra can probably help bridge the gap between a man's sexual response and the needs of a more aggressive partner, but it won't improve the relationship if a woman's sexual aggressiveness is underscored by inner hostilities. An angry relationship is still an angry relationship, with or without an erection, so with or without a potency drug, some compassion and understanding on both sides are vital.

A psychological condition known as paraphilia, or sexual perversion, can cause a person—much more frequently a male than a female—to become totally obsessed with sex. In affected individuals, sex becomes the entire focal point of life, the driving force behind every thought and action. Obviously, this can play havoc with the physical and mental health of both partners, and medical or psychiatric treatment is strongly advised. (I'll discuss a patient with paraphilia a little later.)

Planned or Spontaneous?

In determining their week-to-week, month-to-month sexual habits, each couple makes a choice, either consciously or otherwise, from among three basic options: They may have sex according to a planned, pre-established schedule; they may be completely spontaneous in their selection of times and places for sex; or they may use a combination of planned and spontaneous sexual activity.

For some couples, sex is as predictable a part of their routine as brushing their teeth. On a twice-a-week schedule, for instance, their first sexual episode may take place on Wednesday nights after the late TV news, followed by the "Saturday night special" when they return from a trip to the movies.

For others, nothing is planned more than a few moments in advance, and sex can occur whenever and wherever "the spirit moves them." This system can involve situations ranging from frenetic (dinner guests are due in fifteen minutes) to uncomfortable (on a cold, slippery bathroom floor), even to dangerous (parked on the shoulder of the freeway at 1:00 A.M.), but some couples find that the excitement makes up for the sacrifice and inconvenience.

Clearly, there are pitfalls in both these approaches. Arousal doesn't always occur equally in both partners promptly at ten o'clock every Wednesday night. On the other hand, spontaneous desire is usually felt more strongly by one partner than the other.

Settling into a too predictable pattern may dampen the romantic, adventurous aspects of sex, yet simply being aware that sex is on the agenda for a certain time may help stimulate both partners. Realistically, it's unlikely that both partners will feel the same degree of stimulation when sex is initiated on a totally spontaneous basis. Also, amid the rush and pressures of everyday life, the opportunities for spur-of-the-moment sex may gradually become fewer and fewer.

All things considered then, the third option of combining planned sex and spontaneous sex may be the most advantageous. Flexibility, variety, and compromise are major ingredients in a sound sexual relationship. Couples may also alternate prolonged sexual activity with an occasional "quickie." Even kisses, touches, and other displays of affection that don't lead to actual intercourse can add pleasure and stability to a relationship. To use a food analogy: Sometimes you're in the mood for an elegant five-course formal dinner, but at other times a tasty snack will do.

The "Sexless" Among Us

Thus far in this chapter we've been discussing the quantity and quality of sexual activities as they occur among traditional couples in committed relationships. But it's also appropriate to consider the legions of American men and women who have no such relationships and whose opportunities for sex are greatly diminished or perhaps even nonexistent.

In a society that often seems obsessed with sex, we conveniently tend to forget vast segments of that society that are temporarily— or sometimes even permanently—deprived of sexual expression. Sometimes this results from the person's own decision (to enter a religious order requiring sexual abstinence, for example). Others, such as prisoners or people in sexually isolated occupations, have less choice in the matter.

By far the most prevalent victims of sexual deprivation, however, are those ordinary individuals who are going through life without having a committed relationship—people without regular partners. They number in the tens of millions, and at some point most of us have found ourselves among their ranks, at least temporarily.

In a social system that revolves around couples, single people have special reasons to feel left out or discriminated against when we play the sexual "numbers game." By and large, these men and women have the same basic sexual needs and desires as everybody else, but few acceptable outlets. Many go for months, even years, without sexual intercourse, but does this automatically make them less "normal" than the rest of us? I don't think so.

At the same time, however, growing medical evidence indicates that along with the loneliness and mental anguish suffered by many single people, their lack of sex may also be undermining their physical health. This is especially true in men who abstain from sex, either by choice or necessity. British researchers recently found that middle-aged men who have less than one orgasm per month are roughly twice as likely to die from disease as those who have orgasms more frequently. (This, incidentally, raises serious new questions about the potential health risks of enforced celibacy.)

Obviously, many single men and women are actively seeking suitable mates and committed relationships, and for them the inaccessibility of sex may be only a short-term condition. But for countless others, especially the middle-aged and elderly, the single life can become permanent after the breakup of a marriage or the death of a spouse.

But being without a regular partner doesn't necessarily mean a sexless existence, even for those who shy away from re-entering the dating game. Some people who remain single and avoid committed relationships have also found practical and creative—if somewhat unorthodox—ways of maintaining their sexuality. Many individuals have periodic sexual encounters with another consenting acquaintance without being interested either in a binding romantic relationship or even in sharing any other aspect of their lives.

The Case for Masturbation

For a long time, I've been amazed at how something as widely practiced as masturbation can continue to be so universally condemned. In many quarters, masturbation is still regarded as a despicable form of self-abuse—an ultimate "dirty word."

Generation after generation of adolescent and preadolescent boys have been harshly punished and warned of dire consequences by parents who caught them masturbating. Even after Alfred Kinsey's landmark studies of human sexual behavior nearly a half century ago revealed that the vast majority of males and a large percentage of females masturbate at some time in their lives, the nonsense continued. Youngsters were once told dark tales of masturbation-induced insanity and such bizarre physical symptoms as a wild, shifty look in the eyes, a shriveled penis, and sudden, telltale hair growth in the palm of the hand that performed the vile deed. Some of these misinformed youngsters have grown into adults with lingering feelings of guilt about masturbation. Even in today's more enlightened sexual atmosphere, many people still look upon masturbation as aberrant, indecent behavior, and it remains a taboo subject that millions of adults find difficult to discuss, much less admit to.

The truth is, of course, that most human beings and other primates masturbate, some occasionally, some habitually, and there's no medical evidence that the practice, of itself, causes any physical or mental ill effects. Countless individuals have been conditioned by social attitudes and the reactions of others to feel guilty or "unclean" because of it, but the act itself is neither unnatural nor harmful.

Physiologically speaking, achieving an orgasm through masturbation involves exactly the same process as achieving an orgasm through sexual intercourse. When other sexual outlets are unavailable, masturbation can serve quite adequately as a substitute. Few people would argue that it provides the same quality of satisfaction as sexual intercourse with a partner, but there's no difference in the physical outcome.

While those who play numbers games with sex may not agree, I draw no distinction between masturbation and sexual intercourse. By my definition, both constitute "having sex."

In many instances where one partner's sexual needs and desires far outstrip the other partner's, masturbation can help maintain balance and satisfaction within a relationship. It enables one partner not to place the entire burden and responsibility of sex on the other. It can also provide an acceptable—even healthful—sexual release for people without regular partners.

People masturbate, incidentally, for reasons that aren't always totally sexual. The practice can also relieve stress and anxiety or help a person to calm down and relax before falling asleep.

In doing couple therapy, I've found that it often comes as a shock and surprise when one partner learns that the other uses masturbation as a sexual outlet. Sometimes the person making the discovery also feels threatened by it. A wife who finds out that her husband masturbates regularly may resent his obtaining sexual gratification without her involvement. Although there is no other flesh-and-blood woman involved, she may regard what her husband does as a form of infidelity, and her jealous reaction may be somewhat similar.

Because of this, I don't ask a man to give specific details during couple therapy of the fantasies he may have while masturbating. I strongly feel that a person has no obligation to share those fantasies with his partner.

Fantasies can, however, greatly enhance an individual's sexual experiences, and the same can be said for such erotic materials as books, videos, and sex toys. During individual therapy, therefore, I often find it helpful for the patient to verbalize his masturbatory fantasies. They can reveal a great deal about the inner workings of his mind and provide important indications about how and why his sexual difficulties originated.

Some people can't stand the idea of not being the sole source of their partner's sexual stimulation and excitement. But sexually functional couples in mature relationships are often capable of understanding that sexual stimuli can come from various sources and that if the end result is to increase mutual sexual satisfaction, it makes no difference.

If you have a sexual dysfunction, it's important to overcome your embarrassment sufficiently to discuss the topic of masturbation fully with a health care professional. As a psychotherapist, I always investigate this subject thoroughly with a sexually troubled patient because I've found it to be one of the primary keys to successful treatment. It has a direct bearing on understanding the nature and source of a person's sexual dysfunction.

Here are some of the questions I ask patients most frequently about masturbation, along with a brief explanation of how their answers can shed light on their problems:

Is masturbation a sexual outlet for you?
If the answer is "no," it may reveal a problem with sexual desire or a very restrictive sexual attitude. If the answer is "yes," it leads the therapist to the next question.

Do you notice the dysfunction during masturbation?
If the answer is "no," it indicates that the dysfunction is psychological, rather than organic, in origin.

What is the frequency of masturbation?
Frequent masturbation may be evidence of other problems, such as anxiety or compulsive sexual behavior related to a perversion, such as a preference for pornography over sexual relations with one's spouse.

What do you think about when you masturbate?
Some patients say they don't have any fantasies during masturbation but focus solely on themselves. Others reveal consistent scripts to their sexual fantasies.

Do you rely on erotic literature or films?
If the answer is "yes," I try to determine how the patient decides which book or film to choose. If the material is about cross-dressing, for example, it may indicate a problem with transvestism.

What methods do you use?
The man who tells me, for instance, that he needs the high degree of friction obtained by rubbing his penis with a washcloth (as in the following case study) may be enabling me to understand why he complains of not feeling enough stimulation when he has intercourse with his wife.

The woman who tells me she has masturbated with a vibrator for years provides a vital clue as to why she has difficulty obtaining an orgasm with less intense stimulation.

When Sex Is Obsessive

Like anything else, of course, masturbation is sometimes carried to extremes. When this happens, it can contribute to both physical and psychological problems.

A young woman patient complained to me that her husband of five years never seemed very interested in her sexually. When they did have intercourse—which wasn't often—he was almost never able to ejaculate, and he would often lose his erection. Except for appearing puzzled by what was happening, the woman seemed perfectly normal sexually. She reported nothing unusual about her desire phase or her ability to reach orgasm.

The next step was meeting individually with the husband and obtaining as thorough a history as possible. During this process, I asked him if masturbation was a sexual outlet for him. He dodged the question at first, but finally, with considerable difficulty, he admitted that it was both his predominant and preferred means of sexual expression. He estimated that he masturbated at least once a day on average and sometimes even more often. He also said that he had compulsively used pornography ever since his early teens, a practice that had started when he discovered his father's large collection of erotica.

By now, the reason for this man's lack of interest in having sexual intercourse with his wife was fairly apparent, and when I asked him about his method of masturbating, the explanation became even more clear. He reached an orgasm by rubbing his penis vigorously with a washcloth, and he had become so accustomed to this extreme degree of stimulation that he needed it in order to ejaculate. Vaginal intercourse simply didn't supply the necessary friction.

When I saw the couple together again, the man managed to tell his wife what he had told me, and although she was somewhat taken aback by the revelation, she was also relieved. At least she now understood what was causing the problem and no longer had any need to blame herself.

The larger challenge that still remained was dealing with the husband's severe case of paraphilia—obsessive sexual behavior that focused on his compulsive addiction to pornography. Paraphilia is extremely difficult to treat and may be impossible to cure completely. Many women would refuse to stay with a man whose compulsion had reached such proportions, but with this wife's endurance and support, they were eventually able to resume normal intercourse.

This man suffered from both erectile dysfunction and retarded ejaculation, but by approaching his dysfunction directly—say, with a pill—the physician would have entirely missed the sexual perversion that lurked under the surface and triggered the problem. Limiting the treatment to swallowing a pill would also have enabled the man to continue denying the impact of his perversion on his relationship with his wife. Even with improved erections, he would have continued to expend the bulk of his sexual energies on his perversion, shortchanging his spouse and undermining his marriage.

Pornography sometimes serves a useful purpose in stimulating normal sexual activity, but when it becomes an end in itself, it can threaten relationships and lead to severe sexual problems.

Too Much or Too Little?

For most people, the risk of having "too much sex," in the sense of exceeding limits that could damage one's health, ranges from very remote to nonexistent. Unless a person suffers from paraphilia, the upper limits of individual sexuality tend to control themselves. Men, in particular, can't perform sexually without being sufficiently aroused. If a man's sexual appetite is sated, he simply won't become aroused, yet myths abound about the supposedly debilitating effects of overindulging in sex.

The famous novelist Ernest Hemingway is widely reported to have believed that all men are capable of producing only a certain amount of seminal fluid, and that each time a man ejaculates he uses up part of this finite supply. But this theory has no basis in fact. I know of no health threat or medical condition associated with frequent sex.

On the contrary, recent scientific studies show that too little sex may be far more harmful than too much. Researchers are finding that, rather than sapping human vitality, sex serves as a revitalizing elixir, one that helps keep the prostate healthy in middle-aged and elderly men. Those who continue to have sex at least once a month appear to have a much lower risk of developing prostate cancer. In this area alone, convenient oral medications like Viagra could add years to the lives of sexually dysfunctional men by enabling them to have sex on a regular basis. (We'll deal with this subject more fully in the next chapter.)

Couples of childbearing age who experience difficulty conceiving also may benefit from an accelerated sexual schedule around the time of the wife's ovulation. During this period, a husband whose usual frequency is once or twice a week may want to increase that level to once a day to improve the chances of pregnancy.

Under ordinary circumstances, however, there is no reason for any couple to feel pressured to have sex "by the numbers" or any more or less frequently than suits their personal needs.

Ninety-nine percent of the time, their satisfaction is all that really counts.

Talking to Your Doctor

One of the main goals of this chapter is to try to make readers feel more comfortable about talking to their physicians about their sexual concerns. The introduction of Viagra has stimulated more candid and open sexual discussion among the general public, and my hope is that it will do the same between patients and doctors.

When a doctor conducts a routine physical exam and takes a patient's medical history, the patient's sexuality is one of the most important topics to be investigated. Sexual difficulties revealed as part of this investigation can provide decisive clues about overall health and well-being.

Among the questions your physician should ask are these: Who's the most important person in your life from a sexual standpoint? Do you feel you have problems in your relationship with that person? If so, how would you describe those problems? Are you generally satisfied or dissatisfied with your sex life?

These simple questions and the answers you give to them can change the whole focus of your doctor-patient relationship. They can establish a climate in which it's okay to talk frankly about universal problems that affect every human being. They can make it clear that open discussion of sexual issues is not only permitted in the doctor's office, but actively encouraged. They can also tell your doctor a lot about you and help him or her relate to you on a more personal level—which is very much to your advantage as a patient.

As the discussion progresses, of course, you should be prepared to be asked increasingly specific questions about your sexuality. The more honest you are, the better it will be for both your physical and your psychological health and the quicker you and your doctor, working together, can erase any doubts about what constitutes a normal, healthy sex life for you and your partner.

If your physician fails to ask the right questions, there's nothing wrong with asking them yourself and demanding answers. Physicians who shy away from discussing your sexual concerns might as well hang up signs in their waiting rooms that say, "No sexual discussion permitted here."

In that case, it's time to look for another doctor.

Sex and the Aging Process

Within the first few months after Viagra became available by prescription, several dozen men died while taking the drug. These deaths have received extensive, sometimes exaggerated coverage in the media. As a result, many elderly persons have become somewhat apprehensive about taking Viagra. Some people in the over-sixty age bracket—the very group that stands to gain the maximum benefit from Viagra—may have shied away from the drug, or even from asking their doctors about it, because of these reports.

If you happen to be one of these people, please let me try to put the situation into proper perspective for you.

Certainly an element of risk exists in taking any drug, and that risk may be slightly higher when a drug is fast-tracked by the FDA, as Viagra was. This is why a complete medical exam is essential before a physician writes a prescription for Viagra. The first sixteen deaths reported among Viagra users occurred over a period of about sixty days out of well over one million men for whom Viagra had been prescribed. When considered in the light of other statistics, this figure actually seems quite low. Studies by the American Heart Association have shown the normal death rate among men with cardiovascular disease to range from 185 to 275 per million men in any given month, so the number of deaths among Viagra users doesn't appear to be a cause for alarm.

There is, however, a degree of cardiac risk associated with sexual activity, and since many men with erectile dysfunction also have cardiovascular disease, Viagra may increase their risk of death simply by increasing their level of sexual activity, not because of any danger posed by the pill itself. Unfortunately, the media reports haven't always made this clear, and the implication has been that the drug, rather than underlying disease processes, was causing the fatalities.

Although the FDA's preapproval testing of Viagra wasn't as lengthy or extensive as it has been for some other prescription medications, nothing in the research indicates that the drug is unsafe or that it has any unpredictable ill effect on human health. As mentioned earlier, the only severe health risk associated with Viagra is for persons who are taking other medications containing nitrates, and this risk has been well publicized from the beginning. Every licensed physician in the country should have been well aware of this contraindication long before the death reports surfaced.

Joseph Feczko, Pfizer's top drug-safety official, explained that the death figures were actually "lower than we'd expect, based on the number of prescriptions." Feczko described the company as having a feeling of "reassurance" rather than being disturbed by the figures. "We continue to believe that the drug is safe and effective for its indications and the intended patient population," added FDA spokeswoman Lorrie McHugh.

Despite these reassurances, the hue and cry over the "Viagra deaths" continued. In my area the story kept being rediscovered and recycled for more than a week. It was first reported rather routinely in the newspapers (the *Dallas Morning News* carried it at the top of an inside page in the front section); a few days later, local TV newscasters picked it up; the following week, local radio stations rehashed it yet again. Each time, the story was presented as if it were brand-new, although it was based on the same original—and now stale—information.

Because of the feverish public interest in the subject, I strongly suspect that some medical reporters have, at times, gone in search of another Viagra story every few days. The seventy-year-old New York man whose longtime partner sued him for palimony, claiming Viagra caused him to have delusions of being a young man and sent him out prowling for sex, was picked up by the Associated Press and also got wide media attention. (The drug can change relationships, but it doesn't produce infidelity by itself or of itself. As Dr. Domeena Renshaw, director of Loyola University's Sexual Dysfunction Clinic, told the AP: "If you're a cheater, you're going to cheat—with or without Viagra.")

In some respects, elderly people are more susceptible than younger ones to scare stories in the media. People who are old enough to remember philosopher and humorist Will Rogers generally concur with one of his most often quoted comments: "All I know is what I read in the papers." To many an older person, reading it in the newspaper or seeing it on TV makes it officially true.

As far as is known, Viagra poses no general threat to the nation's elderly. Except for patients with diagnosed heart disease who take a coronary vasodilator drug containing nitrates (see chapter 2 for a partial list of these drugs), there is no documented medical reason for any adult with sexual difficulty—elderly or otherwise—to avoid Viagra. One of the so-called Viagra deaths was caused when paramedics unwittingly gave nitroglycerin to a man with chest pains who had also taken Viagra, so it's important for all emergency medical personnel to be alerted to this danger. In most cases, though, the key for the patient is to have a complete medical evaluation before taking an oral impotency drug. This is true regardless of the patient's age, but it's especially crucial for the elderly.

If you're in your sixties, seventies, or beyond, it's unwise and potentially unhealthy for you to take any prescription medication without having such an evaluation, and Viagra is no exception to this rule.

Do We "Outgrow" Sex?

Because human sexuality is inseparably linked to the reproductive process, it's been widely assumed throughout history that when people move beyond the childbearing stage of life they also "outgrow" their needs and desires for sexual expression. In generations past, various factors combined to make this unofficial rule hold true much of the time. As recently as the early 1900s, "old age" usually arrived much earlier than it does today, brought on by years of arduous labor, faulty nutrition, sketchy medical care, and diseases for which there was no known treatment.

In those days, by the time Ma and Pa hit their fifties, they were often too exhausted from working twelve hours a day and six days a week even to think about a romp in the hay on Saturday night. With no effective means of birth control, many couples began abstaining from sex even before the wife reached menopause, in order to avoid late accidental additions to already large families. Chronic illnesses for which medical science offered little relief robbed many men and women of the energy and interest required for sexual activity.

But that was then, and this is now. Today, tens of millions of couples in their fifties, sixties, and seventies view an active, satisfying sexual relationship as an integral part of their overall quality of life, ranking just behind staying fit and healthy and having financial security. Today, people in this age group are just as conditioned to continued sexual intimacy as their long-ago counterparts were to a mostly sexless existence.

Research conducted in the 1980s by the Center for the Study of Aging and Human Development at Duke University showed that four out of five men aged sixty and over maintain an active interest in sex. Another study, this one of more than 2,800 patients at the California College of Medicine in Irvine, found that half of the men in their fifties and a quarter of those in their sixties continued to have sexual intercourse at least once a week.

It seems, however, that each oncoming generation likes to think of itself as the first to discover sex, and younger people, in particular, still have a tendency to dismiss or take lightly the sexuality of their grandparents' generation. But within the next couple of decades, over-fifty Americans will claim a steadily increasing percentage of the country's total population, and this attitude will most likely change, too.

By and large, I view these as extremely positive developments. Keeping sexual desire and expression in the lives of older Americans can enrich—and, in many cases, actually extend—those lives. And this is an area in which I believe Viagra can make one of its most vital contributions.

Forestalling Old Age

In the not-too-distant past, those who lived to reach retirement and attain the status of "old folks" had plenty of reasons to feel fortunate and grateful. They had to beat some pretty long odds just to achieve those milestones. Think about it: Little or nothing was known about the now-familiar threats to life and health posed by smoking, obesity, high-fat diets, high cholesterol, and physical inactivity. Almost nobody took vitamins, and nutritional supplements were unknown, while such nutrition-related diseases as anemia, pellegra, rickets, and goiter were rampant in many areas. There were no effective medicines to lower high blood pressure, no polio vaccine, no modern surgical techniques, no effective cure for TB, no kidney dialysis.

Over the past half century or so, our knowledge of the aging process has expanded tremendously. Science now knows that "getting old" involves an intricate combination of physiological and psychological factors that are impossible to avoid but that *can* be significantly forestalled—especially for individuals with a healthy lifestyle, good genes, and a positive attitude.

Not coincidentally, our average life expectancy has also increased dramatically during this time—not merely in terms of how long life itself can be sustained but also in terms of how much comfort, enjoyment, mobility, and productivity we can expect during our "golden years." And as the baby-boom generation moves steadily toward what was once considered "retirement age," our national expectations about length and quality of life are likely to rise at an even faster rate.

No generation in history has challenged the status quo as consistently and relentlessly as the baby boomers, and no generation is less likely to settle into its collective rocking chairs and accept the confining traditional concepts of aging. The boomers will fight the aging process every step of the way—indeed, they have already begun—and before the last of them has passed from the scene, they may well have altered society's approach to this whole phenomenon forever.

"I've been amazed by the number of men my age with an interest in [Viagra]," said Dennis M. Taylor, a fifty-one-year-old Helena, Montana, man quoted in *USA Today.* "The fear of impotency must be really pervasive in my generation. We invented the sexual revolution in the '60s, and we are also in the greatest denial about aging."

Fifty or sixty years ago, the situation was enormously different. The vast majority of people beyond the age of sixty or so were automatically defined as "elderly," not just by their families and society in general but by themselves as well. For the most part, they accepted the definition and the role in which they were cast without complaint. Today, the situation has changed completely.

You're Never Too Old

Science is now starting to recognize that sex, like physical activity, good nutrition, and an upbeat outlook, can be a major contributor to a longer, happier life, and that no one who is physically capable of having sex is "too old" to enjoy it and benefit from it.

I've had numerous patients in their mid- to late seventies, and even some who were well along in their eighties, who were still having sexual intercourse on a regular (sometimes surprisingly frequent) basis. As long as a person has the necessary stamina and desire, I see no logical reason to set any upper age limit on sexual activity. I think it's entirely possible for some people to keep having sex up to the age of ninety, one hundred, or even beyond.

Clearly Viagra has the capability to enable countless elderly men and their partners to achieve this type of feat. Some of the greatest enthusiasm for Viagra has been shown by men aged sixty-five and older, and it's in this age group that I think Viagra promises some of its greatest benefits.

I recently treated a retired schoolteacher who had lost his sex life to a prostate cancer operation. He'd tried penile injections without much success, and was ecstatic with the results he obtained from Viagra the very first time he used it. "I take the pill about thirty minutes before my wife and I start getting romantic, and when we're ready for intercourse, we just do it," he said. "It's like it was when we were first married."

I can't imagine any experience that would give an aging man who has been deprived of sexual expression more of a psychological boost or make him feel more youthful. For a person in this situation, Viagra and the other new oral agents for impotency are much more than just an erection-enhancing pill. They can also represent a life-enhancing—and very possibly life-extending—medication.

Orgasms and Longevity

A study reported in the *British Medical Journal* in late 1997 examined more than 900 men between the ages of forty-five and fifty-nine and concluded that those who have regular sex are generally healthier than men who don't. Men in the lowest-frequency group—those who had fewer than one orgasm per month—had a death rate almost double that of those with the highest level of sexual activity (at least two orgasms per week). Even when the data was adjusted for social class, blood pressure, smoking, and heart disease, the risk was still 1.9 times greater for the sexually inactive men.

"Most health messages are telling us to stop doing things, and they tend to have disappointing results," said George Davey Smith, a professor at Bristol University and one of the authors of the study. "Making love may be the only form of exercise for some people, and telling them to do more of something they enjoy could be beneficial."

A great deal more research is needed, particularly among men aged fifty to eighty, on the correlation between regular sexual activity and overall health and longevity. I personally feel that the link will prove to be very real. At present, however, medical experts are engaged in a sort of "chicken and the egg" debate over this question: Is it a lack of sex that predisposes some men to heart disease, or is it the other way around? Do impotency and the resulting absence of sexual activity somehow trigger atherosclerosis, the hardening of the arteries that leads to most heart attacks and strokes? Or does the atherosclerosis occur first, restricting the blood supply to the penis even as it also narrows and clogs coronary arteries?

As yet, medical science has no definitive answer to these questions. We do know, however, that the narrowing of blood vessels characterized by atherosclerosis occurs throughout the body, including in the genitals. So in either case, whether as a marker for coronary disease or as a barrier to the sexual activity that could help prevent it, erectile dysfunction should be considered a serious problem with potentially life-threatening consequences. And even in instances when it doesn't pose a direct threat to survival, impotency can totally destroy a patient's quality of life.

Reasons for Sexual Decline

Unarguably, sexual activity *does* decline with age. The study at the California College of Medicine in Irvine showed that after age seventy, only one man in ten averages having sexual intercourse as often as once a week. This compares to nearly nine out of ten men between twenty and twenty-nine who reported having intercourse at least once a week and about 44 percent of men in this younger age group who had sex three to four times a week.

But many of the factors involved in this age-related decline have nothing to do with sexual function or ability. The main problem is far more likely to be some type of distraction or just plain boredom. In interviewing a group of men aged fifty-one to eighty-nine,

Masters and Johnson found that monotony or repetitiveness in the relationship was the number-one reason given for decreased sexual activity. The second most frequently mentioned cause was preoccupation with a career or economic pursuits.

The next four most often cited reasons were (3) mental or physical fatigue, (4) overindulgence in food or drink, (5) physical or mental infirmities of either the man or his spouse, and (6) fear of failure associated with or resulting from any of the previous causes.

When a long-term sexual relationship grows dull and predictable, both partners tend to lose interest. This is true even with many younger couples, but as the partners age, it frequently becomes a situation that feeds on itself. In this atmosphere, once a man begins experiencing sexual difficulties, he has a tendency to withdraw from sexual activity and use aging as an excuse.

The longer it's been since a man was aroused sufficiently to feel really strong sexual desire, the easier it is for him to convince himself that regular sex is no longer important. Unfortunately, this conclusion is reinforced by a number of persistent—and completely erroneous—ideas about sex and aging.

Old Wives' (and Husbands') Tales

In counseling older patients and their spouses, I often find that one of the first steps is dispelling stubborn myths and baseless superstitions about sexual dysfunction and its causes, and even about deviant sexual behavior as it applies to older men.

Five of the most common of these myths include:

1. Sexual intercourse and ejaculation are debilitating to health and energy, hastening the infirmities of old age and death.
2. One's sex life can be prolonged by abstinence in earlier years and inactivity in later years.
3. Masturbation is childish and/or harmful.
4. Sexual pleasure and satisfaction automatically decrease as a person grows older.

5. Older men who remain sexually active are subject to such sexual deviations as exhibitionism and child molesting. (Actually, exhibitionism is committed mostly by males under twenty-five and is rarely seen after age forty. Child molesters, meanwhile, are more likely to be between their mid-thirties and late fifties.)

Simply explaining away these myths and helping older patients and their partners liberalize their own attitudes can be a big step in eliminating or minimizing sexual difficulties. At the same time, both the patient and the partner must also realize that certain major, unavoidable sexual differences *do* result from aging; the key is to learn to distinguish between myth and fact.

Regular sexual activity can be just as important for older people as for younger people—if not more so—but legitimate differences must be taken into account if the aging couple's sexual relationship is to continue successfully. In many instances, this means altering long-standing lovemaking routines and overcoming resistance to learning new practices that may at first seem awkward, tedious, and even distasteful.

Aging and Sexual Response

Even in the healthiest individuals, the sexual response in both men and women is directly affected by aging. Recognizing and adjusting to these effects is vital to continued sexual fulfillment by both partners.

In men, the most common age-related changes include the following:

1. The need for direct stimulation is greater before an erection can be obtained, and it often takes longer.
2. Pre-ejaculatory fluid is either minimal or absent entirely.
3. The stage of ejaculatory inevitability is briefer and sometimes absent.
4. The amount of seminal fluid is decreased.

5. There is a more rapid loss of erection after ejaculation, followed by a longer refractory period. At times, an erection may be lost without ejaculation.
6. The need and ability for ejaculation at each sexual contact is reduced. Sensations become less concentrated in the genitals and more diffused.

In older women, meanwhile, a corresponding set of changes also takes place, including the following:

1. Vaginal lubrication takes place more slowly, and more direct stimulation is needed. Dryness may persist even with prolonged stimulation, making intercourse difficult unless the vagina is artificially lubricated.
2. The orgasmic phase may be shorter, but the capacity to have orgasms, including multiple orgasms, remains unimpaired.
3. After menopause (or a hysterectomy in which the ovaries are removed), low levels of estrogen can cause irritability of vaginal tissues, pain on clitoral stimulation, or painful uterine spasms during orgasm. Estrogen-replacement therapy can usually alleviate these symptoms.

Becoming a "Dirty Old Man"

It's amazing how few mature men and women have a clear understanding of these age-related phenomena, especially the ones affecting the opposite sex, and the stress they can bring to bear on relationships that were warm and satisfying until the changes began to occur.

In innumerable cases, one partner or the other either fails to realize that something is different or doesn't know how to react to the difference. One partner may want the other to do something he or she has never done before but not know how to communicate these wishes. The message may be garbled in transmission, and even if it isn't, the other partner may not be comfortable with it. Rather than producing mutual satisfaction, the result may be embarrassment, hostility, and stress on the relationship.

"After almost forty years of marriage, my husband's turned into a dirty old man," fumed prim sixty-year-old Helen B. during my first individual therapy session with her. "All of a sudden, Charlie's trying to get me to do things I don't know how to do. Things I don't feel comfortable about."

"What kind of things?" I asked. "Can you be a little more specific?"

She flushed and bit her lip. "Like the stuff you see in those X-rated movies," she said, averting her eyes. "He wants me to fondle his penis for fifteen or twenty minutes before we make love. He claims that's the only way it'll get stiff enough. And for the past few months, he's been wanting us to do oral sex on each other, too."

"I take it from the way you talk that you find this very unpleasant," I said. "Are these things you've never done before—not in all your forty years together?"

She shifted uneasily in her chair, still staring at the floor. "Well, maybe we did once in a while when we were first married and got a little carried away," she said. "But that was a long time ago. Since I went through menopause, I don't even care that much about sex anymore anyway. Sometimes having intercourse is painful for me, so I don't look forward to it much, and having to go through all this stuff Charlie wants to do. . . . Well, it's just embarrassing and disgusting. I think he's perverted."

I spent the next forty minutes or so explaining to Helen what happens to the male sexual response as a man grows older, trying to relate the male changes to the changes affecting her own arousal and orgasm phases, and suggesting how she and Charlie could get more sexually in tune with each other. By the time I was done, she was smiling and shaking her head. She still acted a little embarrassed, but she seemed to have gotten over her anger toward her husband.

"Until just recently, Charlie and I always had a good love life, but we never talked much about it to each other," she said. "I guess we just took it for granted that it'd always stay the same. Then, when it started to change, neither of us knew what to say to the other one about it. We were just fumbling in the dark—in more ways than one."

Rx: Viagra for Two

When I met with Helen and Charlie together, I again went over the points I had covered with them individually, and I encouraged them to be more open with each other about their sexual needs and desires. Then I did something that I've rarely done with a couple in therapy. I prescribed Viagra and suggested that both of them use it the next few times they made love.

I had several reasons for recommending this. For one, I felt certain that Viagra would give Charlie a faster, more reliable erection if he took it an hour before having sex. For another, I had every reason to believe, considering all the available data plus the fact that she was taking estrogen, that the drug would also help relieve the vaginal dryness that was causing most of Helen's problems during intercourse. More important, I doubted that giving Viagra to Charlie alone would improve the situation if Helen was still unwilling to provide the greater direct stimulation that Charlie ordinarily required for an erection. So, to enhance their total sexual experience, I made Viagra available to both of them. (We'll be taking a close look at the overall potential for the use of Viagra by women in chapter 16.)

At last report, Helen and Charlie were doing fine, and I feel totally justified in the course of treatment I followed for them. With counseling, they came to understand why their problem developed and how to deal with it through better, more open, more sensitive communication. Then, with Viagra, they were able to recapture all the physical pleasure and emotional uplift that lovemaking had given them before.

"I feel like I'm on my honeymoon again," Helen confided by

phone a few weeks ago. She also made it clear that she no longer thinks of Charlie as either "dirty" or "old."

"He's the same wonderful man I married forty years ago," she said.

Risk, Reality, and the "Three C's"

As mentioned earlier, the overall risk related to sexual activity by patients with heart disease is very slight—about twenty heart attacks for every million people having sex. But when the sexual activity is with a regular, familiar partner, as opposed to with a new person in a clandestine "one-night stand," the risk drops precipitously.

Some men who may not be diagnosed heart patients could be sufficiently overweight, underexercised, and out of shape to face a slightly higher risk of heart attack simply from the physical exertion of increased sexual activity after taking Viagra. But these individuals could just as easily suffer a heart attack while climbing a flight of stairs or hurrying across a street, and nothing about the drug itself would increase this likelihood.

In my medical opinion, Viagra can be of value for older men and their partners. Properly used in combination with other forms of therapy, it offers hope of painless, dependable relief for much of the age-related sexual dysfunction that impairs mature relationships.

One of the major challenges of the next few years will be to make the nation's health care professionals fully aware of this potential. My hope is that the day will come when no physician will ever again brush off an elderly patient's concerns about sex by saying, "At your age, you shouldn't worry about it."

For many men and women, drugs that effect arousal can permanently erase the myth that loss of sexuality is an inescapable, irreversible part of growing older. They can drive home the refreshing realization that intimacy can survive as long as both partners have life and breath.

But these drugs can't and won't alter character or personality. They won't keep a man at home if he happens to be a philanderer at heart. They won't make love bloom again if one partner erects emotional or psychological barriers against the other.

And they will never replace the "three C's" of a sound, mutually agreeable relationship: caring, communication, and common sense.

15
Who Pays— and How Much?

There are strong and compelling reasons for America's major private health plans and HMOs, as well as Medicare and Medicaid, to cover the cost of Viagra for men diagnosed with erectile dysfunction. I strongly believe that reasonable amounts of the drug should be covered regardless of whether the cause of the problem is organic or psychogenic. As Mariann Caprino, a spokeswoman for Pfizer, told *Time* recently, "Managed-care plans cover conditions like arthritis and allergies because they threaten people's quality of life. That's exactly what we're talking about here [with Viagra]."

I find the comparison between impotency and arthritis highly appropriate. There is no record of anyone having died of either disorder, but the suffering inflicted by either can be intense enough to mar a patient's entire life. If a new drug came along that could quickly erase the symptoms of arthritis in eight out of ten cases, it would undoubtedly be covered immediately by all the big health plans, even at ten dollars per pill. But there has been great reluctance to do so with Viagra.

Much of the insurers' resistance to paying for Viagra seems illogical to me, even from the perspective of the bottom line. Although its price tag sounds unnervingly high to some insurance companies, the per-dose cost of Viagra is actually less expensive than the penile injections and urethral suppositories that most of the health plans already cover. The real bugaboo, however, is the immense popularity of the oral drug. As *Time* puts it, "If even half of the estimated 30 million U.S. men with erectile difficulties started taking Viagra once a week, the cost would approach $8 billion a year. That's terrific news for Pfizer—even a $1 billion drug is considered a blockbuster—but a big burden for the health-care system."

This is yet another reason why physicians *must* use care in prescribing Viagra and why patients *must* be thoroughly evaluated before they begin taking it. Anything that adds to the skyrocketing cost of health care and health insurance eventually stands to hurt everyone. But when a physician conducts a proper evaluation and determines that a patient genuinely needs Viagra, the patient's health plan should pay for a reasonable amount of the drug.

Is It Covered or Not?

For the first few months after the FDA's approval of Viagra, federal officials allowed the various states to decide whether to let Medicaid funds be used to pay for the drug. About a dozen states, including Texas, agreed to let Medicaid patients have the drug, but a dozen others, including New York, California, Illinois, Pennsylvania, and Michigan, rejected coverage. Other states continued to debate the issue.

Later, the Clinton administration moved to require that Medicaid pay for Viagra but to allow states to set limits on the number of pills or prescriptions. Since then, Texas and many other states have set the limit at six pills per month, the same limit established by the Cigna, Anthem, and WellPoint health care programs. Oxford Health Plans and United Healthcare pay for up to eight pills per month.

Either of these amounts is sufficient to meet most couples' needs, and I have no argument with setting some limitations on the maximum number of pills allowed. In my opinion, however, some flexibility is necessary for determining need in individual cases. Both the private insurers and the federal agencies involved should be willing to let qualified health professionals determine the best course for individual patients.

Otherwise, countless patients with real needs could be reduced to ciphers in a mindless, inequitable system. For example, companies might establish actuarial tables on sexual intercourse that show you need less sex (and fewer pills) as you grow older. According to these tables, you may be able to get four pills a month if you're fifty-seven but only three per month if you're fifty-eight. By the time you're eighty, you may be down to one every other month.

And what of all the other variables? Do you get more pills when you go on vacation? Fewer when your spouse dies? More when you meet someone new? Will the actuarial tables cover only frequency of intercourse, or will you be allowed a couple of extra pills for masturbation? Will you be committing insurance fraud if you use Viagra in a way that the insurers didn't intend or if you give a pill to a friend?

These questions may seem absurd, but somebody somewhere is going to have to come up with answers. Unfortunately, the answers may very well mean that someone other than your physician will determine how often you can have an erection.

It also bothers me that several major health plans, including Aetna U.S. Healthcare, Kaiser Health Plans, PacifiCare, and Prudential, don't cover Viagra under their regular plans at present. Aetna offers a separate rider for the drug at extra cost, and PacifiCare and Prudential were reviewing their policies on Viagra as this was written. Kaiser appears to be standing pat on its decision not to cover the drug at all, citing a projected annual cost estimate of $100 million for Viagra—or nearly double the $59 million Kaiser spent in 1997 on all antiviral drugs put together.

I'm further disturbed by the additional restrictions that some insurers impose on Viagra's use. Up to now, for example, Cigna has required that patients have a "pre-existing, documented condition of organic impotence, which is currently being treated by other medical means." Its policy is also under review.

The whole premise of this requirement seems pointless and counterproductive. In the first place, psychogenic impotence is just as real and devastating as organic impotence, and certainly shouldn't be excluded from coverage. In the second place, if Viagra is effective against organic impotence, why should the patient have to continue treatment by "other medical means"—and why should a health plan pay for that other treatment?

"Viagra represents a whole new spectrum of drugs, the likes of which we haven't had to deal with before," says Dr. Joseph Berman, chief medical officer for Anthem Inc. The drug falls into a gray area somewhere between medical necessity and lifestyle enhancer.

Few patients or doctors would protest an insurer's decision not to cover cosmetic surgery or a drug that stimulates hair growth, but paying for a drug that treats sexual dysfunction is more problematic, Berman says. Anthem decided to cover Viagra because it pays for other forms of therapy for erectile dysfunction and, he adds, because it's "a very good treatment."

A Dose of Common Sense

Clearly, the health insurers are struggling with the whole issue of Viagra and other similar drugs—and with good reason. A commonsense approach, however, could benefit the companies as well as the people they insure. Why, for instance, should the insurers continue to pay out large sums for such expensive treatments for erectile dysfunction as surgical implants, which can cost thousands of dollars, but refuse to cover oral medications? At most, Viagra will cost an average of sixty to eighty dollars per month, while allowing a quality of life that surgical implants could never provide.

Even so, I anticipate that many patients will end up paying out of their own pockets for Viagra while the insurers attempt to drive down costs and increase profits. It may take a concerted lobbying effort and legislative pressure by concerned citizens groups to secure adequate coverage for erectile disorders. But HMOs are already under heavy fire in Congress from both major political parties on charges that they have denied and delayed care for millions of patients. In this atmosphere, it may be easier for the public to win concessions on Viagra and similar drugs.

And instead of bowing their necks on Viagra coverage, the insurance companies might make creative use of the Viagra issue to attract corporate clients. ("Subscribe to our plan and we'll throw in six pills a month as a bonus.") Employers, too, will play a key role in whether or not their employees are covered for oral impotency drugs. Some employers may offer rich benefits packages including such drugs as an attractive fringe benefit for employees. Others may elect to go the cheaper route. Still others may give employees both options.

Undeniably, it's a complex issue, one of the thorniest yet to face the managed-health-care industry and one that isn't likely to be settled any time soon. When other new oral impotency drugs hit the market, and if and when the FDA eventually approves Viagra for women, the situation will be complicated still further.

It goes without saying, however, that any attempt to exclude Viagra and other oral impotency medications from Medicaid or Medicare coverage would be a terrible injustice to untold millions of elderly and indigent Americans. With the states exercising a large measure of control over Medicaid, the disadvantaged face the greatest obstacles in obtaining effective impotency treatment. The large public-sector hospitals and clinics to which disadvantaged patients must turn for treatment are traditionally more concerned with life-threatening conditions than with conditions that merely affect quality of life. To some extent, this is understandable, but it still isn't fair.

As the *Dallas Morning News* observed in a recent editorial, "The Viagra debate shouldn't be about sex, income or gender. Like so many other drugs, Viagra provides patients with a prescription drug to treat an established medical condition and improve the quality of life. After all, that's the purpose of medicine." I couldn't agree more.

Access to Specialists

Rationing of the medication—often in ways that are unjustified and arbitrary—is only one part of the problem facing patients in managed-health-care plans as they try to obtain relief from sexual dysfunction. (The term "managed-health-care plan" is actually a misnomer in most cases, by the way. What these plans are intended to do is manage health *costs*, so "managed-health-cost plan" would be a far more accurate term.)

The other half of the cost-cutting equation is limiting the patient's access to specialized medical care, and this leads to other, less obvious questions that also must be considered. Will your plan allow you to consult a specialist who knows something about sexual medicine? Can you, for example, go directly to a urologist for an erectile problem? Under most plans, the answer is "no." You must first go to a "gatekeeper," a general physician who has a financial disincentive to refer you to a specialist. If a GP sends patients to specialists too often, he or she may be dropped as an approved provider. But how much knowledge and experience does the GP have in diagnosing and treating sexual dysfunction? The usual answer is "little or none."

Any physician, of course, can write a prescription for Viagra. But before you congratulate yourself on your impressive new erection, consider the fact that you may also be the proud owner of an undiagnosed brain tumor.

This is the first time I can recall in more than thirty years as a practicing physician that patients are being barred by their insurance companies from consulting the health care providers with the most education, training, and experience in diagnosing and treating a specific illness. The situation is changing in some states where consumer groups are pushing for greater accessibility to specialists, but in far too many cases, the doors to the specialists' offices are still being kept locked by the insurers.

Meanwhile, if you and your partner should need sex therapy, you really have a problem. Most managed-care companies are very unsophisticated when it comes to psychotherapy of any kind, since they regard talking to patients as something that practically anyone can do. Don't be surprised, therefore, if you're referred to the least-trained, least-experienced psychotherapist available, since this is the cheapest route for the insurer. You probably won't get the psychodynamic understanding, relational dynamics, or behavior therapy offered by a health care professional with heavy experience in treating sexual disorders, but that's not the company's problem.

What do you do in this situation? If there are indications that the cause of your dysfunction is organic—such as no morning erections and no erections with masturbation—you need a thorough workup. Don't settle for a Viagra prescription and a pat on the back. Demand to see a urologist. If there are signs of relationship problems or other functional factors, insist on seeing an experienced psychotherapist. And don't be afraid to ask the physicians to whom you're referred for credentials relating to their training and experience in treating sexual disorders.

The point is that patients *do* still have rights, even under managed-care plans and HMOs. You may have to talk a little louder and be a little more persistent than you once did in order to exercise these rights, but the results can be worth the extra effort.

16 Women and Viagra

From the moment Viagra appeared in our midst, women have been every bit as emotionally caught up in the phenomenon of the drug as men have, and in some cases even more so. Amid the maelstrom surrounding the drug's public introduction, feminine reaction to it has run the gamut of emotions, from hostility and ridicule to hopeful optimism and unconcealed curiosity.

Indeed, much of the initial clamor for Viagra was generated by women who were aware of their partners' sexual problems, believed the drug could help, and either urged their men to ask their doctors about it or called the doctors themselves. Many physicians reported that an amazingly high percentage of the calls they received about Viagra during the early weeks of its availability came from women, and my own experience bears this out.

At the same time, however, there has also been a groundswell of decidedly negative reaction from a large segment of the female population. Many women remain dubious, suspicious, even fearful about the overall consequences of the drug. They are concerned about a male tendency to oversimplify complex relationships by thinking that a hard penis can solve any sexual problem.

To some extent, these female misgivings are justified, although there is growing evidence to indicate that men increasingly share women's concerns about intimacy. I'll talk more about that a little later, but the point I want to make now is that in the not-too-distant future I foresee a significant number of women taking Viagra. In fact, while almost all the public and media attention has been focused on Viagra as a "male potency pill," thousands of women have already begun using the little blue pill to enhance their own sexual experiences. And this is just the beginning.

In the meantime, however, a large and highly vocal segment of American womanhood has gone on the attack where Viagra is concerned. As sociologist John Gagnon, co-author of the book *Sex in America*, explains, many women don't believe that "good sex will come from a pill," and they also don't see Viagra producing intimacy, expressive moments, or a caring attitude toward the other person.

In an interview with *USA Today*, Gagnon summed up female negativism toward the drug when he added, "All this pill does is make the penis harder. Wow!"

Pessimism and Putdowns

Dr. Ruth Westheimer, probably the nation's best-known sex therapist, spoke for many women soon after Viagra became available when she told *Time*, "Even if a man has an erection from floor to ceiling and can keep it that way for an hour, it will not be pleasurable for a woman if he is not sexually literate. There has to be an education process to go with this drug."

Best-selling author Gail Sheehy, who recently published a new book about male menopause, also took a rather skeptical, pessimistic tone in discussing Viagra. Six months before its approval by the FDA, Sheehy wrote an article in *Newsweek* warning that "men face a larger challenge to their virility and vitality than can be 'cured' by any magic bullet."

Then, a month after the drug appeared in pharmacies, Sheehy claimed in an interview with *USA Today* that many men were already calling their doctors to express dissatisfaction with Viagra with such comments as "I could have spent my $10 on a pizza [instead]." Although this reaction undoubtedly did occur in isolated instances, the statement leaves a false impression, since far more men have been pleased than disappointed with Viagra.

"There is a lot of 'couples work' that has to be done to make [Viagra] work," Sheehy concluded. I totally agree, and this has been the essence of my approach to using the drug. But if Sheehy is implying that women are somehow being excluded from this process, I definitely *don't* agree.

Postfeminist social critic Camille Paglia used Viagra's approval to voice an especially caustic putdown of the modern American male in a commentary on the Internet. "Viagra might even be vital to our national defense," she said, "since it is highly unlikely that the last two generations of mewling, puling milksop males have the strength or will to resist a serious military threat to the United States."

Earlier, in a *Time* interview, Paglia had said: "The erection is the last gasp of modern manhood. If men can't continue to produce erections, they're going to evolve themselves right out of the human species. I want men to re-examine, really re-examine why they need this pill. Because they do need it; they need it right now."

A *New York Times* column by Maureen Dowd was more good-natured but equally sardonic. "Women already think men are led too much by their anatomy," she wrote. "If Pfizer's rivals are smart, they are looking for the Viagra antidote. For each woman who celebrates Viagra, there's another who has nightmares about her 62-year-old husband undergoing a satyric transformation and chasing 21-year-old interns, his desk littered with empty Viagra bottles. . . . As men know, women like to think they're special. With Viagra, women will never know for sure whether it's their own allure or just chemically enhanced blood-vessel function."

Not Just a "Guy Thing"

These comments all contain some food for thought. But classifying Viagra as purely a "guy thing" and using it as fuel to heat up the war between the sexes hardly seems justified—especially since women may soon be taking the drug as freely and frequently as men.

Within the next few years, I fully expect the FDA to alter its initial interpretation that Viagra is indicated for use only by adult males and to officially extend its use to women. But in the meantime, there are no legal restrictions against women taking the drug or against physicians prescribing it for them. As this is written, it's impossible to estimate how many women have actually used Viagra, but conservatively speaking, I think the figure could run into the tens of thousands.

For some months, Pfizer has been funding the same type of double-blind, placebo-controlled clinical trials with women that scientists previously conducted with men, and with strikingly similar results. In studies involving five hundred women in England, the pill has passed all Phase I safety tests required by the FDA, and Phase II testing is well under way. Dr. Frances Quirk of the Pfizer research team is helping develop a questionnaire for women in the British studies that will shed new light on the sexual psychology of women and their attitudes about sex, as well as on female sexual dysfunction.

What the studies have shown so far is that Viagra produces the same increased blood flow to the female genitals as it does to the male genitals. In the presence of sexual stimulation, this leads to increased vaginal lubrication, which is the female equivalent of an erection.

Up until very recently, little medical attention had been focused on the sexual difficulties experienced by many women during and after menopause. Like men in their fifties, sixties, and beyond, women in these age groups were widely assumed to lose sexual interest and capability as part of an inevitable aging process. Since physicians usually didn't ask older women about their sexual complaints, and since women are far better at "suffering in silence" than men, everybody just sort of looked the other way and ignored the problem.

But as more information emerges about sexual problems among

older women—and as more women enter the over-fifty age groups—the true scope of female sexual dysfunction related to menopause is rapidly being revealed. I strongly suspect that if thirty million American men have some degree of erectile dysfunction, at least that many women have some degree of lubrication dysfunction.

What Menopause Means

There is good reason why menopause has long been referred to as the "change of life." It triggers several changes in a woman's body, many of them unpleasant, painful, and distressing. But while the hot flashes, night sweats, headaches, insomnia, nervousness, depression, and irritability may be more immediately noticeable, no change has more far-reaching impact than what often happens sexually during and after menopause. Usually, these physical sexual changes coincide with a time of heavy psychological pressures that are causing the woman to reassess her whole life and identity.

"There are so many changes going on for women especially at this age," says Dr. Michael J. Daly, professor of obstetrics and gynecology at Temple University Medical Center, in an article in *Medical Aspects of Human Sexuality*. "From the time she gets up in the morning and looks in the mirror at herself, she is reminded of the aging process. When there are no children to get off to school, she is reminded of it. Her husband is less romantic and possibly less interested in sexuality so that intercourse is less apt to occur."

In this atmosphere, the woman feels insecure and apprehensive, and her husband's reaction often doesn't help matters. In referring to how this might happen in a traditional marriage, Dr. David M. Reed, professor of psychiatry at the University of Pennsylvania School of Medicine, describes it this way: "She is suddenly alone again with the man she married thirty years ago. But he has his nose in the *Wall Street Journal,* and he doesn't look up and say hello to her anymore at breakfast, except on the way out of the house, because he is terribly busy making the next move in his career."

When this happens, a woman's entire view of her own sexuality and her ability to attract a man can be severely damaged. She may react by having an affair, not to pacify her libido but in a desperate search for the affection she's missing at home, to prove to herself that she's still needed and wanted and that she can still be loved and attract a man.

At this same crucial point, however, decreased lubrication and accompanying loss of sensitivity to sexual stimulation can effectively destroy the sexuality of many menopausal and postmenopausal women. Inadequate lubrication can cause discomfort or pain during intercourse, nullifying sexual pleasure and the ability to obtain an orgasm.

These are facts that have largely been obscured amid the recent furor over male impotency, but we now know that a high percentage of women—particularly those past age fifty—also suffer from sexual dysfunction. Dr. Irwin Goldstein, a Boston University urologist and veteran sex researcher, found, for example, that more than half of the female partners of impotent men also reported having sexual performance problems of their own.

Estrogen-replacement therapy can be of some benefit in relieving vaginal dryness and discomfort, but estrogen has no influence on the arousal phase or overall sexuality in women.

"Estrogens given to the estrogen-deficient female will improve the turgor and the epithelial structures in the vagina, and make the vagina more usable as the receptive organ for the penis, but not necessarily influence the female's sexual response," says Dr. Alvin F. Goldfarb, professor of obstetrics and gynecology at Jefferson Medical College. "In my opinion, sexuality reflects the total well-being of the middle-aged woman. . . . I do not feel that I can personally solve the problems of frigidity in the menopausal and postmenopausal woman by giving her estrogens. . . . I think most of the problems of sexuality in the menopausal patient are referable to problems of general health, problems of emotional outlook, and problems of family life."

Viagra to the Rescue

As with male sexual dysfunction, sexual problems in women may result from a confluence of many factors, and medical treatment of other conditions may be necessary. There are also serious disease processes that can affect female sexuality, and it's important to rule these out before concentrating on treating sexual dysfunction. But for millions of women suffering sexual distress as a direct result of menopause, Viagra offers hope for a normal sex life in middle and old age.

From all indications thus far, the drug has vast potential for helping women whose sexuality has been impaired by the "change of life" to lubricate normally and to enjoy a better response to stimulation. And in women with medical conditions that prevent them from taking estrogen, Viagra is already proving extremely beneficial in increasing lubrication and improving the quality of intercourse. The drug may also benefit women who have problems with the arousal phase because of fatigue, depression, or reactions to drugs.

In short, Viagra's effect in women appears to be similar to its effect in men. Additional research is needed to produce conclusive proof of its safe general use for female sexual problems, and until the current trials are completed, physicians should exercise care and caution in prescribing Viagra for women. As of now, the drug's total effect on the female body hasn't been established. There's no proof, for example, that it won't hinder fertility in some way or cause birth defects, so it definitely should be avoided by pregnant women.

Nevertheless, the little blue pill shows every sign of being a true "equal opportunity" medication that offers unique benefits for both sexes.

"I Want to Be a Guinea Pig"

While the British clinical trials continue, other studies of women and Viagra are being carried out in the United States with grants provided by the American Foundation for Urologic Diseases and other organizations. In late April 1998, about a month after the FDA approved Viagra, one hundred of the nation's top research scientists gathered in Bethesda, Maryland, to pose a fundamental question: "What is the female problem that Viagra would solve?"

First of all, it's vital to understand that women *do* have a problem and that it may often be compounded by the fact that the affected women themselves fail to realize it. A man's erectile dysfunction is embarrassingly obvious, both to himself and his partner, while a woman's is much less apparent because she can still perform. Yet as many as 50 percent of adult women questioned in some surveys admit that they have lost interest in sex or have difficulty becoming aroused.

Just as they do in men, narrowed blood vessels and aging can also interfere with genital blood flow in women, giving them a numb sensation during intercourse and making it difficult for them to be sexually stimulated. Viagra has proved especially beneficial to women whose sexual function has been impaired as a result of surgical removal of the ovaries.

Laurie Kline, a Baltimore hairdresser, participated in a Viagra study conducted at the University of Maryland, Baltimore, by Dr. Jennifer Berman, a urologist at Boston University School of Medicine. After taking her first pill, Kline reported having the first orgasm she had experienced in the entire five years since her ovaries were removed. For obvious reasons, she was totally sold on the drug. "It was really wonderful," Kline said. "It was like it used to be, maybe even a little bit better. It seemed like my body was back like it was before."

While Pfizer spokesmen officially discourage the "off-label" use of Viagra by women until further testing is completed, thousands of women from coast to coast have shown a willingness—even an eagerness—to accept whatever risk may be involved.

At age thirty-nine, Robin Lyles, another participant in the Baltimore study, had also undergone a complete hysterectomy, and immediately afterward she had noticed that her sexual performance declined sharply. When invited to try Viagra, she jumped at the opportunity. "If it's something that's going to help me the way I need it to help me, I'll take the risk," she said. "I want to be a sort of guinea pig."

Lyles and Kline are far from being alone in these sentiments. According to Berman, "hundreds of women" asked to be placed on a waiting list in hopes of taking part in the Baltimore study.

Many other such "guinea pigs" have also reported dramatic results with Viagra. In a separate study in Minneapolis, fourteen of sixteen women who had Viagra prescribed for them by Dr. Mario Petrini, an obstetrician-gynecologist, experienced improved sexual response. Most took the drug in combination with testosterone to boost their libido. In Chicago, six women took the pill alone in a study at Loyola University Medical Center, and three reported enhanced arousal.

As acclaim for Viagra has grown—with such luminaries as former Republican presidential nominee Bob Dole; his wife, former Transportation Secretary Elizabeth Dole; and even Pope John Paul himself singing its praises—more and more women have been impressed with the legitimacy of the drug.

Sex clinics from Manhattan to Miami report being deluged by calls from women whose interest in Viagra is purely personal, and dozens of women have been quoted on the Internet as saying that they and all their friends "can't wait" to try Viagra.

"Almost every woman my age wonders if sex could be better," said a fifty-five-year-old nurse who participated in a small independent Viagra study. "Now I know that, for me, at least, the answer is 'yes.' "

The Meanings of Intimacy

It's no secret that countless American women, including many who consider themselves happily married, are dissatisfied with their sexual experiences. Several recent surveys and studies have substantiated this dissatisfaction.

But in my experience, women patients rarely complain specifically about their husbands having trouble with erections. What I hear far more often is that the woman is dissatisfied with some aspect of the intimate relationship.

One long-term study reported in the *Journal of Personality* examined the sexual attitudes and satisfaction levels of more than 1,200 men and women. It showed that, over the past twenty years, both sexes came to regard intimacy as increasingly important as a source of personal fulfillment. Surprisingly, perhaps, the men in the study felt almost as great a need for intimacy, on average, as the women. What was different was how men and women experience intimacy and the needs it fulfills for each sex.

For women, emotional intimacy tends to lead directly to happiness with their relationship roles. If intimacy is satisfying, erections and orgasms assume less importance. For men, on the other hand, a sense of closeness is not as strongly related to their satisfaction with personal relationships as it is to their sense of certainty about the world in general. In other words, intimacy can serve as a springboard of confidence for a man, allowing him to achieve and excel in his outside endeavors. This isn't a new idea, of course. It's pretty well captured in the old adage "Behind every successful man stands a good woman." In an updated version for the 1990s, we could say, "Every successful man has a good relationship with a woman."

It's interesting to note the differences in what men and women perceive as intimacy. For women, the term can be defined as shared feelings. For men, the most satisfying intimacy is experienced when the couple shares enjoyable activities together.

In my practice, it's not unusual to see couples in which the wife wants a greater closeness with her husband. In such circumstances, I frequently hear women say, "If he loved me, he'd know what I need. I shouldn't have to tell him."

My approach is to support both partners. I encourage the woman to be more specific and to put her needs and wishes into words so there will be no confusion. Invariably, though, she fears that by doing so, she runs the risk of being rejected by her husband. Typically, she worries that he may interpret what she says as criticism and that this may cause a negative reaction on his part. So these issues, too, have to be explored and resolved.

At the same time, I also try to help the man understand his difficulty in sharing his feelings with his wife, and I urge him to accept the risk of sharing. He invariably perceives himself as vulnerable, and at this point, he feels threatened by communicating his feelings, so this is also explored.

I see what happens in my office during these sessions as a microcosm of what happens hundreds of thousands of times each day in society at large. If both parties are willing to state explicitly what their needs and fears really are, then it contributes to greater understanding between the partners—and to greater closeness. This doesn't always have to take place in a physician's office, however. It can happen at home, too, if couples are willing to be open and caring enough toward each other.

I don't believe that Viagra or any other pill will, of itself, create closeness, warmth, and intimacy between two people. Many men manage to convince themselves that if they had firmer, more dependable erections, their relationship with their partner would automatically improve. My experience tells me that this is seldom, if ever, true, and I have yet to see this idea borne out in my clinical practice.

I can state unequivocally that I have *never*—not once in more than thirty years of sexual counseling and therapy—encountered a woman patient who believed that a lack of erections was the only problem in her relationship with her partner. This is why I believe that any therapy focused only on getting an erection ignores larger, more crucial issues. For the sake of the relationship, these issues must be addressed.

In this context, I can certainly empathize with the initial negative reaction to Viagra by many women. But at the same time, women should understand that this drug is much more than just an "erection pill" for men and that attempts to make it a "gender issue" are shortsighted and self-defeating. Properly used, it *can* help enhance intimacy as well as improve the physical aspects of sex.

Help for Special Problems

Viagra also stands to benefit countless thousands of female patients with special medical problems that affect their sexuality. In fact, it's already being hailed as a godsend by some of these women who have had the opportunity to try it.

I prescribed Viagra recently for a forty-year-old female patient who was being treated for depression. She was taking one of the newer antidepressants, which have fewer adverse sexual side effects than the older ones, but it caused her to become overagitated, so I had to put her on one of the older drugs. The medication helped her depression considerably, but it also interfered with her arousal phase and vaginal lubrication.

"I have almost no interest in sex," she reported, "and I get no pleasure at all out of intercourse. The last time my husband and I tried it, I just had to tell him it was too uncomfortable."

Two weeks later, after taking Viagra three times, the woman had an entirely different story to tell. "It's unbelievable," she said. "I feel like I'm seventeen again—and my husband *acts* like he's seventeen, too."

Antidepressants are just one of several prevalent causes of temporary lubrication and arousal problems. Many women with chronic allergies or sinus problems who take antihistamines to dry up their runny noses fail to realize that these over-the-counter remedies can dry up their vaginal fluids as well. A connective-tissue disorder known as Sjögren's disease also interferes with normal lubrication in all areas of the body, including the vagina, mouth, and eyes.

As mentioned, the most common cause of lubrication difficulties is probably a shortage of estrogen in menopausal and postmenopausal women, but women who have had their ovaries removed may experience this problem even earlier in life. Regardless of the cause, once the body stops producing estrogen naturally, most women can take replacement doses of the hormone to keep it at a desirable level. But for some, hormone-replacement therapy represents a greater potential health threat than not having enough estrogen.

I counseled one patient recently who had precisely this kind of problem. Within the past four years she had undergone both a hysterectomy and a radical mastectomy of her left breast due to breast cancer. Because estrogen replacement increases the risk of breast cancer, she had been warned by her oncologist to avoid it at all costs. Yet the absence of estrogen stemming from her hysterectomy had left this patient with severe vaginal dryness that made sexual intercourse painfully impossible.

I felt that her situation was tailor-made for Viagra. I had no hesitation at all about prescribing it, and the results couldn't have been more gratifying.

An hour after taking her first pill, the patient became aroused and lubricated normally during foreplay with her husband. A short time later, they had intercourse for the first time in months, and the patient had her first orgasm in more than two years.

"All systems are 'go' again," she told me cheerfully on her next visit. "These pills are utterly incredible."

Bridging the Sexual "Gap"

One of the greatest differences between the female and male sexual response lies in the timing involved. This is also one of the principal causes of sexual dissatisfaction in women. It relates directly to what they perceive as male preoccupation with the physical act of sex and disregard for the emotional closeness and intimacy that women value.

When it comes to instinctive sexual behavior, men and women simply aren't on the same schedule most of the time. On average, men are much more easily and quickly aroused than women, and unless some effort is made to adjust the schedule, the male sexual response may run its full course while the woman is still in the early stages of the female response.

This is why a man may think a woman is "cold" or "turned off" when, in fact, she simply hasn't had time to warm up yet. It's also the reason a woman may characterize a man's lovemaking routine as "a couple of kisses, a few quick thrusts, a groan, and a snore."

Women have the capacity to become just as fully and forcefully aroused as their male partners, and once their excitement phase peaks, they can remain at that plateau for a long time—far longer than most men. Unfortunately, millions of women are abandoned at this plateau each night by men whose sexual energy has come and gone while the women's was still building. While their men lie satiated and sleeping, they are left without the sense of intimacy for which they yearn, and also without an orgasm. Can anyone blame them for feeling cheated?

It takes the average woman much longer to reach an orgasm after the initiation of intercourse than it takes the average man. This frequently leaves a significant time gap separating them from mutual sexual fulfillment—a gap that is very real and very disturbing for many couples. I know, however, that the gap can be bridged to give both the man and the woman a more pleasurable, satisfying sexual experience. All they have to do is remember the two "magic words":

Slow down!

Adequate foreplay is critically important to sexual satisfaction in most women. Studies have shown that when foreplay lasts for at least twenty minutes prior to beginning actual intercourse, about nine out of ten women are able to reach orgasm. But when foreplay is cut short, this figure plummets.

How the Clitoris Works

The literal "nerve center" of the female sexual response is the clitoris, which is the female counterpart to the male penis. The clitoris has the same number of nerve endings as the penis, and like the penis, it becomes engorged with blood during sexual stimulation.

Many women are unable to reach an orgasm during sexual intercourse, and the reason is invariably insufficient clitoral stimulation. Ordinarily, the clitoris becomes hooded during intercourse and inaccessible to direct touch by the penis. Therefore, it has to be stimulated by indirect pressure.

This is why manipulation of the clitoris during foreplay is often essential. If the woman is to achieve an orgasm during intercourse, she must usually be "on her way" before intercourse is initiated.

The man can also enhance the woman's sexual pleasure and increase her chances of reaching orgasm by using what is known as the "coital alignment technique" during intercourse. This involves altering the motions of the man's penis and using his weight to apply added pressure to the clitoris. With the man above the woman, he moves upward so that his weight is positioned over the woman's pubic area, rather than supporting his weight with his arms and legs. And instead of the usual in-and-out thrusting, the partners move together in a kind of circular motion, which prolongs the man's erection and facilitates the woman's orgasm.

Sufficient clitoral stimulation usually requires both patience and initiative on the man's part, but there is no surer way to enhance his partner's sexual pleasure or fulfill her need for closeness and intimacy.

A Pill for Each Partner?

At some point in the future, when a couple wants to have a really satisfying sexual experience, it may become common practice for both a husband and wife to routinely swallow a pill an hour or so before intercourse.

Assuming that Viagra is found to be fully safe and appropriate for general use by women, this scenario seems quite conceivable to me. Within a few years, it could be happening millions of times each night all over the country.

Frankly, for partners who want to refresh themselves sexually and rejuvenate committed relationships, I see absolutely nothing wrong with this concept. Even at twenty dollars a pop, it could be worth it.

There are valid reasons to believe, in fact, that the use of Viagra by both partners could eliminate many of the current female concerns about the drug. There would be far less likelihood of producing the type of one-sided sexual experiences, heavily weighted in favor of male erections and male egos, that some women fear.

Whereas better sexual functioning by just one partner could actually serve to destabilize a relationship, sharing Viagra would ensure that both partners shared equal benefit. It would be far less likely for one partner to feel shortchanged or that he or she was merely being used as an object for the other's gratification. Experiencing greater mutual satisfaction, partners might feel much less temptation to stray outside the relationship.

And maybe—just maybe—a drug whose introduction has stirred up a lot of age-old animosities between the sexes could end up pointing the way toward more peaceful and pleasurable coexistence.

What the Future Holds

To a large extent, this book has been about Viagra, but it was never intended to promote any drug or family of drugs. One of its goals has been to endorse a healthy, reasonable way of using those drugs and other forms of sexual therapy to build the best possible relationships. Another has been to present as objective an overview as possible of what is happening today in the complex realm of human sexuality.

Now it's time to take a few speculative glimpses at what the future may have in store.

In the short time since Viagra entered our vocabulary, two fundamental facts have emerged about American society in the late 1990s: (1) there are far more sexually troubled men than many of us realized; (2) for the first time ever, we have a simple pill that can do something about it.

Likewise, there are two distinct aspects of the Viagra phenomenon. There is the drug itself, unquestionably the most effective oral agent yet devised for sexual dysfunction. Then there is the supercharged atmosphere of sexual awareness engendered by the drug. In this atmosphere, many more men have become more open about their sexuality than ever before. They are saying, in effect, "Hey, I just realized I may be part of a problem that affects millions of other guys—but now I can be part of the solution, too."

The "Aspirin of Sexuality"

As a drug, Viagra is of vast, indisputable importance. On average, it quickly, painlessly, and predictably improves erections in about eight out of every ten men who have taken it. And while there are no definitive figures as yet on the exact percentage of women users who experience improved lubrication and/or heightened response to sexual stimulation, indications are that Viagra can help a sizable percentage of women.

And yet, much as it may warrant the designation of "miracle drug," Viagra is *not* a cure-all. It will *not* restore sexual performance in 40 to 50 percent of men whose impotency is caused by serious organic disease processes. These men will still have to rely on pumps, injections, or implants, or live without sexual intercourse.

It also won't solve the many personal conflicts and personality problems that hinder sexual performance. By itself, it can't save a floundering relationship, and it may, in fact, "grease the skids" for already troubled marriages where affection has been eroded by bitterness.

Viagra isn't the only drug of its type, either. It's merely the first in an entire new family of drugs for treating sexual dysfunction. Within a short time, other prescription medications offering similar results will also be on the market. Some may be less effective than Viagra, while others could offer even greater advancements in treating sexual dysfunction.

Viagra may be more widely remembered in years to come than the drugs that follow it because of the precedent it set, just as aspirin is remembered today as the first effective over-the-counter pain reliever and fever reducer. We now have any number of painkillers that are more effective and have fewer unpleasant side effects than aspirin, but aspirin was still the first, and it remains the standard in its field. Long after Viagra is forced to share the sexual-dysfunction drug market and the billions of dollars it generates in sales each year, it may still be regarded as the "aspirin of sexuality."

Viagra's role as a social catalyst, however, is even more important, and its influence transcends the drug itself. In the future, its appearance may well be remembered as the cutting-edge force that created a whole new public attitude about the sexual problems that are so prevalent in modern society and about the entire subject of sex in general. Its appearance has become such a watershed event that we may one day come to designate everything that happened prior to April 1998 as "before Viagra" and everything since as "after Viagra."

Issues Physicians Face

The thorniest social issues surrounding oral impotency drugs must be faced head-on by every physician attempting to treat sexual disorders, and these issues aren't likely to go away. On the contrary, I think they'll be with us for decades to come, and they may well intensify as time goes on. At least one major lawsuit has already been filed against Pfizer. Others will undoubtedly follow, both against the drugs' manufacturers and the physicians who prescribe them.

Even without the impending threat of legal wrangling, the moral and ethical considerations for conscientious health professionals are almost endless, and so is the potential for conflicts. Should a physician prescribe an oral agent to men or women whom he knows to be involved in extramarital affairs? What reservations may be felt by some doctors in prescribing the drugs for gay men? Men who are being treated for AIDS are often impotent, so what about them? Does their capacity for contributing to a death-dealing worldwide disease epidemic outweigh their need for effective treatment? Is the physician justified in denying oral agents to such men?

What about men who suffer from both paraphilia and erectile dysfunction? These men are often emotionally immature, and their marital relationships are often threatened, but will improving their sexual performance strengthen their relationship with their spouses or merely drive the men deeper into their sexual addiction? Will it make them less dependent on their perversion for sexual excitement—or more?

Viagra is contraindicated for convicted sex offenders, but questions about exceptions to the rule will inevitably arise. What about offenders who have served their sentences, entered committed relationships, and are closely monitored by parole boards? If they develop erectile dysfunction that seriously impairs their marriages, should they be allowed a few pills under strict supervision and with the understanding that any abuse of the privilege would mean withdrawal of the drug? I would still say "no," but in isolated individual instances, other physicians might decide otherwise.

Even the matter of prescribing Viagra for women raises major ethical questions at present, since much remains to be learned about its effects on females. No doctor should knowingly prescribe it for a pregnant woman, at least until much more extensive testing has been completed, but some pregnant women might conceal their condition in order to get the drug. Physicians must take extreme precautions to avoid such possibilities.

It's impossible to overstate the need for careful and complete evaluation of every patient who asks for Viagra for any reason. I'd much prefer to see the medical profession adopt an overly strict approach to sexuality drugs, rather than go in the opposite direction.

At the same time, however, every patient has the right to a second opinion. If your physician has moral or ethical concerns that prevent prescribing Viagra or similar drugs for you, he or she should tell you straight out. You then have the right to ask for a referral to another physician, who may not share these qualms.

Altering Our Life Patterns

A few scientific milestones—the discovery of penicillin, the development of the smallpox and polio vaccines, the pasteurization process for protecting food from bacteria—have benefited the health and longevity of billions of human beings. Other triumphs of science, however, such as the invention of gunpowder and the splitting of the atom, have led to untold human agony and pushed the world to the brink of destruction.

But again, the importance of these discoveries goes beyond the suffering and death that they directly either caused or prevented. They also set in motion momentous changes in the way we live our daily lives and how we relate to each other and the world around us.

Whether Viagra, along with the birth-control pill, merits a place on this short list of landmark scientific achievements is still to be determined. Perhaps a mere "sex pill" doesn't belong in the same ranks with lifesaving antibiotics and vaccines. Yet Viagra has already changed the way we think and act as a society with regard to the most elemental and emotionally charged of all human functions, and that change is likely to become more profound as time goes by.

As I write, Viagra is legally available only in the United States, Mexico, Morocco, and Brazil, but by the time you read this, it will most likely have been approved in Colombia, South Africa, and Thailand, and by early 2000, Pfizer expects it to be available worldwide. This means that Viagra's societal influences will soon be felt in every corner of the globe.

At this moment, it's impossible to say what the future impact of the Viagra phenomenon will be. It will likely take several decades before scientists, sociologists, politicians, physicians, and educators are able to assess its overall effects and make an objective judgment. By then, of course, there will be no way to undo those effects. For better or worse, they will have become an ingrained part of human civilization. For better or worse, they will touch all of us.

This much is certain, however. Viagra has already shed more light on the once forbidden area of sexual function than any medical discovery since the dawn of time. And as important as the drug itself is, its social and medical side effects stand to be even more far-reaching. Viagra's appearance has thrown open the door to frank discussion and enlightened study of human sexuality in a way that no scientific development has ever done before.

The fact that it has also caused some men to act like fools and sent some women into a rage does nothing to negate its potential for rewriting the behavioral future of America and the world.

The Best of All Worlds

Let's look ahead for a moment to, say, thirty or forty years from now. By then, we should have enough medical and social experience with Viagra and its spin-off effects to formulate some meaningful measurements of their total influence on our way of life.

In a best-case scenario, here is part of what the "Viagra age" could spawn by the midpoint of the twenty-first century:

We could see a cease-fire in the perpetual war between the sexes as men and women embrace a new openness and candor in dealing with sexual and personal difficulties. By improving intimacy and allowing couples to keep romance alive in their relationships, even in the face of advancing age and serious health problems, sexuality drugs could lead to a sharp drop in the divorce rate, especially among the over-forty population.

We could also see a couple-oriented approach being universally used by all physicians in treating sexual problems in either partner in a relationship, and counseling required along with drug therapy. Often both partners may be coordinating their ingestion of oral drugs for sexual dysfunction.

With comprehensive new medical school programs, physicians may become much more knowledgeable about sexuality and sexual problems than they are in the 1990s, no longer telling patients they are "too old to worry about sex" and understanding that nobody is too old. Couples could routinely continue to have regular sexual intercourse well into their eighties and nineties, and some centenarians might still be sexually active. This development could help increase the average American's life span by several years.

Because of the demonstrated relationship between an active sex life and increased life expectancy and the treatment and prevention of life-threatening disease, Viagra-type drugs may be approved by all major health plans with coverage based on the individual needs of patient and spouse. No harmful side effects from long-term use of these drugs would be found when they are taken within these limits. Competition among the various brands of medications and the introduction of generic alternatives could cut the price per pill to a fraction of today's cost.

The federal government and all fifty states could enact strict laws carrying heavy criminal penalties for improper sale or distribution of sexuality drugs to convicted sex offenders. Parental consent would be required before the drugs could be prescribed for anyone under age eighteen.

Sexual dysfunction would no longer be a subject steeped in shame and embarrassment. In fact, questions about sexual function would be among the first things most physicians would ask their new patients. Sexual problems would be easy to treat and recognized both as early-warning signs of potentially serious diseases and as reliable guides for treating them. In short, when it comes to sexuality and sexual relationships, Viagra's legacy could create the best of all possible worlds.

Sounds great, doesn't it? But now let's look at the other side of the coin and a possible worst-case scenario.

Opening Pandora's Box

By, say, 2035 or so, the Viagra phenomenon could become a Pandora's box of social and medical calamities for the Western world.

A booming black market could make sexuality drugs as accessible to the public as marijuana. To combat it, Congress might consider legislation to make the drugs over-the-counter products. Meanwhile, a catastrophic new sexual revolution may have swept the country, fueled by a youth-cult mythology even stronger than the one that once surrounded Spanish fly. Despite repeated reassurances from the medical community that Viagra-style drugs have no aphrodisiac properties, young singles of both sexes could become convinced that the drugs contribute to arousal as well as enhancing the physical sex act, leading them to pop the pills indiscriminately.

Physicians might no longer attempt to screen patients before prescribing sexuality drugs or to monitor or counsel patients who take them. Medical societies could justify this ultralenient approach by pointing to the easy availability of the drugs and the fact that those prescribed by doctors at least met accepted safety and dosage standards, unlike black market versions produced by the billions in illegal labs.

Most younger people might avoid marriage or committed relationships, preferring to "graze" from partner to partner in search of the mythical ultimate sexual experience. Among over-fifty couples, few marriages would last until the death of one partner or the other. The rest would end in divorce or permanent separation. An atmosphere could prevail in which men and women in their seventies and eighties casually traded partners at "Viagra parties" and middle-aged swingers abandoned their mates for "Viagra weekends" at exotic resorts.

We can even envision hordes of motherless and fatherless children roaming the streets and jamming emergency shelters. The products of casual liaisons between sex partners who were virtual strangers to each other, these children might simply be abandoned. And with few remaining stable marriages, the chances of their being adopted or finding a foster home could be practically nil.

Laws to keep sexuality drugs out of the hands of serial rapists and child molesters could be largely ignored. If so, the rate of sex crimes in major urban centers could jump to several times what it is in the 1990s.

Sexually transmitted diseases could reach epidemic levels, and the annual death rate from AIDS could skyrocket. Habitual daily users of sexuality drugs could find themselves at high risk of severe health problems of which we know nothing today. "Viagra addiction" could also become a serious problem affecting millions of people.

I could go on, but I think you get the picture.

Pluses and Minuses

While I don't pretend to be a soothsayer, and our attempts to predict the future often miss the mark by a mile, something very similar to either of the scenarios above could theoretically happen. A more likely projection for Viagra's future, however, would be a mixture of good effects and bad.

Our experiences with the birth-control pill are an example of just such a "mixed bag" of pluses and minuses. Today, more than thirty years after the introduction of "the pill" and the beginning of the sexual revolution that swept the nation in the 1970s, debate still rages over the results.

To some extent, the pill may have helped stem the population explosion that many economists of the 1960s feared would soon deplete the earth's vital resources, and it has undoubtedly prevented tens of millions of unwanted pregnancies. It has allowed women to enjoy a sense of sexual freedom and sexual equality that they never had before. Used wisely and carefully, it has also allowed adequate planning for and desirable spacing of children in many families.

But on the negative side, the pill is closely associated with a surge in promiscuity and infidelity, sexually transmitted diseases, and broken relationships. Some sociologists cite it as a factor in sending the divorce rate soaring to record high levels and, ironically, in placing more children in single-parent households than ever before. It has increased the risk of stroke in women and even contributed to the deaths of some of its users.

For middle-class America, the pill has largely lived up to its promise of smaller, better-planned families. But in the view of some social critics, its greatest failing has been its inability to reduce the birth rate among those who might have benefited the most—the poor and underprivileged. Its cost, combined with religious prohibitions and limited access to health care, has denied the pill to most of the world's disadvantaged women. Consequently, although the birth rate in the industrialized nations has leveled off, it continues to soar in developing nations, as well as among our own lower economic classes in the United States.

From the standpoint of pure scientific effectiveness, the birth-control pill is a resounding success. Its record for preventing conception isn't 100 percent, but it comes close. Taken as directed, it interrupts the natural ovulation process, so that no matter when or how often a woman has intercourse, her egg can't be fertilized by her partner's sperm.

But this applies only to the pill itself, not the social phenomenon that it set in motion. To date, the record on that score is, at best, a blend of positives and negatives. Even after thirty years, the jury still hasn't reached a conclusive verdict.

Viagra's unfolding story could well follow this same pattern. The drug itself is overwhelmingly successful in doing what it's supposed to do: make sexual intercourse easier and more enjoyable for the vast majority of people who take it. But how beneficial or detrimental its overall influence may be on our most hallowed social institutions remains to be seen.

The principles used by health care professionals in prescribing the drug and the maturity with which it is used by the public will play a major role in determining how high or low Viagra's marks will be three or four decades down the road. So will the firmness with which reasonable rules and legal limits are applied to its availability and the quality of consumer-education programs formulated to deal with it.

Totally Different Purposes

Despite certain parallels between Viagra and the birth-control pill and the frequent temptation to compare the two, it's important to remember that the basic purposes for which they are intended and used are totally different.

The birth-control pill is strictly a preventive measure that negates a normal physical process and has potential implications on human health. The sexuality pill, on the other hand, is a medicine that effectively restores a natural physical function and thereby relieves a specific medical condition. One interferes with natural physiology, while the other facilitates it. One is a legitimate treatment, the other a mere convenience.

There are other crucial differences as well. No woman in her right mind could find any reason to take more than the prescribed dosage of birth-control pills. But some men will inevitably feel that if one Viagra pill produces good sex, then two or three might produce super sex and be tempted to experiment accordingly. (This type of overdosing on Viagra could produce serious as-yet-unforeseen ill effects.)

Then, too, birth-control pills are usually taken by younger women in relatively good health, while the typical Viagra user is an over-fifty man with a likelihood of having at least one chronic medical condition.

Few users of birth-control pills are inclined to loan a few to a friend. But I already know of any number of men who have shared their supply of Viagra with their curious buddies. "Every guy wants to see how the stuff acts on him and then compare experiences with someone else," explains one sharer.

Meanwhile, the psychological differences involved in using the two drugs are even more profound than the physical differences. As we've repeatedly seen in this book, sexual dysfunction is frequently produced by psychological factors alone or by psychological factors working in tandem with physical factors. Even when the immediate cause is physiological, many cases of sexual dysfunction are complicated by underlying emotional conflicts within the relationship.

A decision to use birth-control pills, on the other hand, is usually based on purely practical considerations, rather than emotional ones. For whatever reason, a woman wants to avoid or delay having children, so she decides to take the pill. In doing so, she develops no ongoing dependence on the drug, and her partner is neither physically nor psychologically affected by her decision. Later, if conditions become favorable for childbearing, all the woman has to do in most cases is stop taking the pill.

The Easy Way Versus the Right Way

What it boils down to is that far more care and caution than is required with birth-control pills must be exercised with Viagra and the other oral impotency agents—both by those who dispense them and by those who swallow them.

Physicians should be careful to explain the proper use of any drug and point out its potential side effects before prescribing it. I believe this is good practice even with a drug as widely used as the birth-control pill, where technically nothing beyond a routine pelvic exam is needed, and no real counseling is necessary. But in my estimation, Viagra should never be prescribed until after the patient's overall health has been thoroughly evaluated. And if psychological factors are contributing to sexual dysfunction, the patient—and his partner, if he is in a committed relationship—should receive thorough counseling.

This isn't necessarily the easy way or the way that most patients would prefer, but it's the *only* right way.

The rubber-stamp approach taken by some physicians in prescribing Viagra not only is reprehensible but also sows the seeds for catastrophic consequences in the future. The medical profession's tendency to routinely prescribe a pill for every complaint must stop with Viagra. Otherwise, doctors will be making themselves accessories to an epidemic of uncontrolled abuse.

The temptation among men to use Viagra for cosmetic effect or as a sex-toy gimmick is widespread and growing. But there is no evidence to support the idea that men whose erections are already rigid and reliable will have their sexual powers and abilities enhanced by the drug. For 99 percent of these men, taking a ten-dollar erection pill will be as pointless as stuffing their money down a rathole.

However, some men *will* be boys, as the saying goes, and some who are fully functional sexually will go to great lengths to obtain Viagra. The only effective way to prevent chronic nationwide abuse is for physicians to maintain tight controls on the drug and a strict set of criteria in prescribing it.

At best, there will be a flourishing black market, fed by smugglers who can purchase large supplies of the drug abroad, then easily carry it across our open borders with Mexico and Canada. If the demand justifies it, some drug runners may even find Viagra a more profitable commodity than marijuana or cocaine. But most of the potential for massive nationwide abuse lies in the hands of America's own physicians and pharmacists. Unless they take a responsible approach, that potential will undoubtedly be realized.

Not a Universal Panacea

As this is written, Viagra has been on the market for only a few months. Within this brief time frame, I've already seen it accomplish remarkable results in a number of patients whose relationships were genuinely helped by it and whose partners were as pleased with it as the patients themselves. But I've also seen Viagra fail, both in producing erections and in improving relationships.

As anyone realizes who has read exaggerated newspaper accounts of "Viagra-charged" octogenarians chasing thirty-year-old women and demanding sex, the drug is *not* a universal panacea. My own observations have been of a less sensational nature, but I do know of at least two or three Viagra users whose wives are now in the midst of divorce proceedings. Clearly, Viagra wasn't enough to salvage their marriages, not even when it was combined with counseling and couple therapy. I also have some diabetic patients and some with prostate cancer who haven't been able to overcome their impotency with Viagra. They must continue to rely on the clumsy, distasteful alternatives that many people presumed would be rendered obsolete by Viagra.

Releasing any new drug into the general population entails hidden risks and pitfalls that no amount of controlled clinical studies can reveal. Despite the fact that people have died while taking Viagra, I feel the drug is as safe as any on the market. Yet, at present, we have no way of knowing all the long-term effects of taking Viagra on a regular, ongoing basis for, say, ten or fifteen years. Only the passage of time can reveal the truth. Also, we can't yet know the complete range of its possible harmful interactions with other drugs when taken together over a prolonged period. In the meantime, the only safe approach is moderation and good sense.

Despite the drug's almost limitless potential for problems and misuse, I remain excited and optimistic about the Viagra phenomenon. But I have no intention of letting my optimism reduce my commitment to caution in prescribing it for my patients. If every American physician embraces this same commitment, sexually dysfunctional men and women will benefit immeasurably from the new class of oral impotency drugs, and our social fabric and cherished institutions will be strengthened, not weakened.

But if a huge segment of the medical community adopts a careless, quick-fix approach to the sexuality drugs, our civilization could be shaken to its foundations.

Medical professionals must instead take the lead in educating the public on the safe and proper use of oral impotency agents. We must counteract the tendency of many patients to trivialize their erectile disorders or resort to reductionism—that is, reducing their sexual problems to minor status in their own minds.

Now that there is an effective oral agent for impotency, many patients will be seduced into believing that a simple solution will always be possible for an extremely complex problem. I see this happen every week, in patients with the most devastating types of psychiatric illness who present their entire problem as a mere chemical imbalance. It's too easy for people in search of "magic bullets" to regard erectile dysfunction in the same light—merely as a deficiency of nitric oxide in the genitals, for instance. What I and other therapists must help them understand is that the release of nitric oxide, which is essential to male sexual performance, is only the final step in a long, complicated journey that leads through psychological jungles, social wastelands, and biological forests. And a misstep in any of these regions along the way can disrupt that delicate final step.

You and your physician need to put erectile dysfunction within the context of your entire internal mental life, your most important relationships, and your overall biological function. Not to do so demeans your sexuality even as it trivializes your problem.

In one way or another, a revolutionary new era in human sexual relations lies before us. Many of us may never know for sure whether, in the final analysis, the net results of this revolution turn out to be good, bad, or somewhere in between, because it may not run its course in our lifetime. Nevertheless, we Americans of the late 1990s are destined to play a key role in the eventual outcome of this new revolution. Even as it shapes us, we will also shape it through the way we relate in the months and years ahead to a small blue pill—and to our own sexuality.

The world will eventually move beyond Viagra, the pill. But it may never move beyond the fundamental social changes that the pill has set in motion. What we and Viagra sow today, our grandchildren are sure to reap tomorrow.

Index